Perspectives in Nursing
1987–1989

*based on presentations at the
eighteenth nln biennial convention*

Pub. No. 41-2199

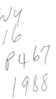

National League for Nursing • New York

ISBN 0-88737-384-4

Manufactured in the United States of America

CONTENTS

v

THE HEALTH CARE
ENVIRONMENT

GUIDING THE FORCES
OF THE HEALTH CARE REVOLUTION

Joseph A. Califano, Jr.
Senior Partner, Dewey, Ballantine, Bushby, Palmer & Wood
Washington, D.C.

A revolution in the American way of health care is underway and it's likely to be as far-reaching as any economical and social upheaval we've known. The stakes are high. Who gets how much money out of one of America's top three industries? Who suffers how much pain and for how long? And who gets the next available kidney, liver, or heart? In short, who lives, who dies, who pays, and who decides?

The revolutionary forces at work are profound. Science is serving up biomedical breakthroughs that hold the promise of remarkable cures for illness and the threat of unacceptable causes of death. The graying of America presents a burgeoning elderly population that consumes the most expensive high-tech medicine and that already strains our capacity to provide adequate medical and nursing care. In law and religion, our judges, ethicists, and theologians are confounded by the Pandora's box of medical discoveries. They must reexamine questions as fundamental as when life begins and when it ends. Concerned about waste and inefficiency, major buyers of health care, including governments, corporations, and big unions, are changing the way many physicians, hospitals, and other providers are used and paid and they're reshaping financial incentives to encourage patients to use the health care system judiciously.

Guiding this revolution is a delicate and treacherous business; there is so much of value to preserve. The American way of health care is nothing short of miraculous. The miracles are everywhere—vaccines that have virtually eliminated most childhood diseases, technology that makes possible vital organ transplants, machines that scan the body and brain and do the work of the heart, and pharmaceutical inventions that remedy everything from headaches and depression to

---

Reprinted by permission from *Nursing & Health Care.* (1987). *8*(7), 401–404.

hypertension and epilepsy. We have conquered diseases that have killed millions over many centuries and we have expanded life expectancy beyond the wildest expectations of just a generation ago. We have an abundance of specialists and an abundance of hospitals.

However soaring costs threaten to deny even affluent Americans access to the miracles we have come to expect. In fact, the billions we've spent have not given millions of our fellow citizens access even to basic health care. Medicine's high priests, the physicians, have said once too often that only they know what to prescribe, where to treat us, and how they should be paid. Corporations, unions, governors, mayors, legislators, and all the presidents of the United States since Lyndon Johnson have attacked profligacy in the American health care system and tried, in one way or another, to cap hospital costs.

There are some signals of change. Hospital admissions, lengths of stay, and occupancy rates have dropped in the last three years. The Medicare program, once predicted to go broke by the end of this decade, looks solvent until the middle of the next. Americans are smoking less and reducing their levels of cholesterol. These early results of our health care revolution are promising, but we must recognize that the revolution is just beginning and that ominous signs still exist. For example, the consumer index (CPI) rose 1.1 percent in 1986, while medical care's component of it rose seven times as fast—7.7 percent. And for the first part of this year, it's still rising substantially faster than the CPI.

THE CHRYSLER STORY

At Chrysler Corporation, where I serve as a board member, we've adopted the kind of hard-nosed health care consumer attitudes that have moved the health care revolution forward. From 1983 to 1985, Chrysler cut health care benefits spending by $100 million. The company now spends about $50 million less per year than it would have without its cost-cutting initiatives. At the same time we're providing better quality health care for those enrolled in our benefits programs.

To accomplish this feat, Chrysler took on a massive, unchecked system that consumed colossal sums of money. In 1981, when Lee Iacocca asked me to join the Chrysler Corporation Board of Directors, he told me Chrysler's health care costs alone could block the company's recovery. He asked me to set up and chair a health care committee for the board—an innovation in American business at the time. The two of us and United Auto Workers' President Doug Fraser served as the first committee members because, as Iacocca put it, the three of us have done more to create the problem than any three people in America: I helped invent and administer Medicare, Medicaid, and other major health care benefits for the United Auto Workers; and Iacocca had agreed to virtually every one of Fraser's demands.

The first thing our committee did was ask, "What are we getting for our health care dollars?" We discovered that we didn't know. Chrysler was then spending about $300 million a year for health care and had no idea what it was buying or from whom. We didn't know who the efficient suppliers were. We had no quality controls. We didn't have the slightest idea of what kinds of health care services our employees truly needed. So, our first step was to get the facts. We took a 30-month snapshot of our health care purchases. We examined more than 67,000 hospital admissions records and more than $200 million in charges. We catalogued each incident of inpatient and outpatient care for every Chrysler employee, retiree, and dependent.

Here's some of what we discovered for the year 1981:

- Lab tests for Chrysler-insured beneficiaries totalled some $12 million. That comes to more than five tests for every man, woman, and child insured.

- Blue Cross/Blue Shield payments per dermatologist were more than double those for the average practitioner, and 25 percent greater than the average payments for chest surgeons. Dermatologists took more of the Michigan Blues' health insurance dollars than any other specialists.

- In Detroit, the cost for patients' average hospital stays at the six largest acute-care hospitals ranged from $3,028 up to $6,077—a 100 percent spread. And the variances were just as wide in the fees physicians charged for the same services and in the kinds of tests and X-rays they prescribed for the same diagnoses, even when they practiced on the same floors of the same building.

- Physicians' post-admission visits to hospitalized patients turned out to be the single most costly procedure Chrysler paid for that year—a total of $4 million.

- Prescription drugs, particularly those with a high street value such as Librium and Valium, were widely abused.

TAKING ACTION

With these findings, the committee went into action. We wanted Chrysler-insured beneficiaries to become alert consumers—to scrutinize their medical bills—so we started a program called One Check Leads To Another. Under this program, Chrysler shares refunds for overcharges with employees and retirees who find them. We substituted equally effective generic drugs for high-priced brand names, established general health maintenance organizations, and mounted health promotion programs with cost-cutting potential. For example, it now costs 50 percent more for optional life insurance for Chrysler employees who smoke than for those who don't smoke. We also tried to move in on areas of major abuse, such as podiatry services.

The big savings, however, came from our efforts to do away with unnecessary hospitalizations. These efforts began with an education campaign to change the way our employees viewed hospitals. We spread the word that hospitals are settings to stay out of, places to go for treatment only when all else fails.

Secondly, we spoke directly with administrators at hospitals with high profiles of unnecessary admissions or needlessly long stays. Here's an example. We had a team of physicians examine our Michigan hospital expenses for nonsurgical low back pain treatment. They found that two-thirds of those hospitalizations at the eight Detroit area hospitals with the most admissions, as well as 85 percent of the total number of days those patients spent in the hospital, were inappropriate. At three of the hospitals, there was not a single appropriate admission. The admissions, it turned out, were largely for bed rest, which is both safer and cheaper at home. We confronted the physicians and administrators with our findings, and they were a little testy at first. But in the first six months following our intervention, those eight hospitals reduced admissions for low back pain by 64 percent. We found the same thing, incidentally, this past year as we began to study other sites in St. Louis and Newark, Delaware, and we're talking to hospital administrators and physicians there.

Finally, and perhaps most importantly, we introduced a screening program for patients planning to go into hospitals. Chrysler will not pay for hospital stays in nonemergency, non-maternity cases unless the need for admission is confirmed by a second, independent practitioner's opinion and a specific length of stay is approved for reimbursement, both prior to the admission date. If the admitting physician believes the stay should be extended beyond that period, he must go to Blue Cross in advance, explain why, and get approval.

Here's how the screening program works. We're informed of a physician's decision that his or her patient needs some kind of elective surgery, and we relay this information to one of the nurses who run this program under the supervision of physicians. The nurse reviews the patient's profile and the length of stay requested and, based on her studies and on the formulas we have, indicates whether she agrees or not. If the patient's physician agrees with the nurse's assessment, that's the end of it. If the physician disagrees, then we contact another physician who is an expert in the area in which the surgery is taking place to investigate the matter.

We're also introducing special preferred provider programs. Chrysler will now pay in full for certain health care services only if they are performed by practitioners in the preferred provider program. These services include eye care and podiatry, and we're planning to add substance abuse, psychiatric, and outpatient radiology services as well as medical equipment, such as prostheses, to that list. Employees and their physicians will have a strong financial incentive to use these providers; using others will mean stiff copayments.

To cut our costs for lab tests, we recently requested bids from reputable laboratories in the Detroit area and chose the lowest. The highest of the bidders came in at 25 percent below what we had been paying. Our employees will be reimbursed for the full cost of outpatient lab tests when their physicians use our designated labs.

These are substantial achievements for Chrysler and other health care purchasers who are trying to take steps to bring about better quality health care for less money. However, the toughest work lies ahead. Where are we headed? What is likely to happen over the next several years?

I think we'll see at least 400,000 unnecessary hospital beds eliminated. And within 10 years, we'll probably need about half the hospital beds we have today. Closing hospitals, as you well know, is hard labor. Everyone admits there are too many hospitals beds in America, But they're all in somebody else's city or congressional district. But the advantages of reducing the number of beds and consolidating facilities are not limited to cost-savings. We now know that by concentrating surgical procedures in fewer locations, we improve medical care. We know, for example, that a patient is seven times more likely to die during a coronary bypass operation in a hospital that performs only 100 such operations per year than in a hospital that performs 350.

We will see extreme and unwarranted variations in the practice of medicine brought to light and scrutinized. A 1984 Massachusetts survey of surgery rates indicated startling variations in medical practice there. Residents of Hingham, Massachusetts were four times more likely to have their gall bladders removed than residents of Holyoke with the same symptoms. Residents of Fairhaven, Fitchburg, and Framingham were 15 times more likely to have their tonsils removed than were residents in other parts of the state. And a study last year of 4.5 million Medicare beneficiaries revealed that the erratic practice of medicine is a national phenomenon. The researchers looked at 123 medical procedures and found that, for 67 of them, patients in the highest rate areas were at least three times more likely to be subjected to them than were patients in the lowest rate areas. Patients in the highest rate areas were eleven times more likely to get a hip operation; six times more likely to have a knee replaced; three times more likely to have coronary bypass surgery; and five times more likely to have a skin biopsy. These variations had no apparent relationship to patients' health statuses.

The cost-savings possibilities are phenomenal. By adopting more conservative surgical practice styles, physicians could easily reduce by 40 percent the money spent on hospitals alone—that translates to $60 billion a year.

I think we will see more competition in the field as purchasers of health care become better informed. And if there are going to be a variety of delivery systems, it is imperative that we have available all kinds of information about health care; what hospitals and doctors charge; how successful they are in treating different types of patients; what kind of diseases they treat most frequently; and how often they resort to such therapies as surgery and potentially addictive drugs.

I think we'll also see a healthy loosening of physicians' tightly held grip on the practice of medicine. Medical technology now makes it possible for nurses to provide treatments such as chemotherapy, dialysis, and intravenous therapies and feeding in homes, nursing homes, and in physicians' offices. There are a number of tasks once reserved for physicians that nurses can perform, including examining, diagnosing, and treating many wounds and sprains as well as common respiratory ailments. Physicians should use their power over the practice of medicine to incorporate the realities of modern technology into it, to eliminate obsolete work rules, and to allow other health professionals and paraprofessionals to provide the many medical services they are capable of performing just as competently as physicians and far less expensively.

We also have to overhaul the medical malpractice system. The cost of malpractice insurance is paid not by physicians and hospitals but by all of us, as taxpayers and patients. Last year, premiums exceeded $4 billion, and billions went for unnecessary tests ordered by physicians to defend themselves from litigation. I believe states should limit the amount of recovery to modest payments for pain and suffering and strongly link damages to the cost of health care, to replacing loss of income due to inability to work, and to disability costs. Contingent legal fees should be sharply reduced.

We must devise and adopt case management systems to cope with high-cost cases, and I think nurses will play a major role in these systems. When Chrysler started the in-depth analysis of its health care data, analysts discovered that 3.4 percent of our employees accounted for 43 percent of the company's hospital payments. When we looked at these high-cost cases, we found that they often involved life-style-related diseases, and that there were situations in which care could have been provided far more effectively, and more humanely, if someone had been watching the store. We found many cases in which employees or retirees went to the hospital, spent anywhere from one to twelve weeks there, and then died, without receiving treatment other than palliative measures to relieve pain. Obviously, these patients were sent to the hospital to die. This was due, in part, to the fact that Chrysler had no program of hospice care and didn't, at that point, provide adequate reimbursement for home nursing care. We now do. And we have nurses managing these cases.

Substance abuse cases, particularly alcoholism cases, were also on Chrysler's high-cost list. These individuals would go to the hospital for detoxification, go to a 30-day residential program, and then come back to work. All of that cost Chrysler somewhere between $20,000 and $25,000. Six months later, they'd be back in the hospital again. Neither our foremen nor our supervisors were adequately trained to watch alcoholic employees and help them stay on the road to recovery after treatment. We're changing that, too.

We need sophisticated health promotion programs. Each of us can do more for our own health than can any physician, any hospital, any machine, or any drug. Heart disease is a prime example. It is our country's number one killer. Many Americans believe that coronary bypass surgery, hypertension pills, transplants, and other modern miracles are largely responsible for the decline in deaths from heart attacks. They could not be more wrong. Since 1970, Americans have witnessed a dramatic 25 percent drop in deaths from coronary heart disease primarily because of their improved eating habits and their efforts to stop or not start smoking.

Hard-nosed bargaining by business and government officials and competition among providers will bring down health care costs and give us a much more efficient system. But the pressure of vigorous competition leaves little space to provide "Robin Hood" care for the elderly, the poor, and the unemployed, even with well-intentioned cost shifting. In such an environment, government must protect vulnerable individuals and assure them access to medical services or they will be squeezed out of the health care system. It would be tragic if we finally got a health care system efficient enough to provide high-quality care for all of our citizens and we failed to satisfy this obligation in social justice.

Catastrophic care coverage is another crucial issue in the revolution. I believe we should have such a plan, but that we have got to be careful not to tilt care back into the most expensive sector—the hospital. Congress should not craft a catastrophic plan that provides billions for hospital care for the elderly, but no funds to permit them the dignity of passing their final days at home, in a hospice, or in a nursing home. To achieve this, I think any catastrophic health care proposal should stipulate that any person eligible for expensive, high-tech hospital care be permitted to choose home, or other less-institutional care and be guaranteed the same full reimbursement.

Nurses' critical roles in the health care revolution must encompass schools. It is my belief that we should return to a system in which every school has a nurse who can pinpoint high-risk students, such as children of alcoholics, and make sure that preventive action is taken early.

At the other end of the spectrum, it is also imperative that we emphasize the importance of and the dignity inherent to caring for our nation's rapidly expanding elderly population. Everyone knows what a mother does for her children when they're ill, but most Americans have no sense of, and attach none of the same kind of dignity to, the work that thousands of nurses do every day to care for elderly people. And few Americans have even begun to think about the unfunded health care liabilities looming as the graying of America comes to pass. For the Fortune 500 companies alone, those liabilities exceed the value of all their assets and, in fact, exceed the size of the national debt of $2 trillion.

Nowhere is America faced with more opportunities and with more danger than in the area of health care. We're at the dawn of the first four-generation society in the history of the world. That dawn can be the start of a brilliant era in which great grandparents pass on a rich living inheritance of love and wisdom to their great grandchildren, or it can be the start of a frightening era of death control. In *The Painful Prescription,* Henry Aaron and William Schwartz argue that, like Great Britain, we will soon ration health care in America. We've always had rationing, of course, related to individuals' economic wealth. But, with Medicare, the government becomes the health care gatekeeper for those who use and need the acute care system most. Bluntly put, Uncle Sam will soon be playing King Solomon with your father and mother and mine—and with you and me. Without the most energetic pursuit of efficiencies, we will soon face a world without kidney dialysis for people over 55, a world without hip operations or artificial hips for those over 65, and a world in which eligibility for expensive anti-cancer therapy will be based on statistical assessments of success. We'll be faced with a world of bureaucratic death control.

That's not a pleasant vision for the future. But in Great Britain, that future is now; that's just about what they do today. We in America are fortunate because we still have time to avoid that fate. We can learn from Britain's experience. We are a far more productive society, and the central fact about health care and costs in America is that we can do something about them. We can't create heaven on earth, but we have the capacity to provide quality care for all at a reasonable cost. We can shape a competitive system of excellence and motivate doctors and hospitals to provide less expensive care while motivating patients to stay healthy. We have the moral depth to face the bewildering ethical issues our scientists pose with their ingenious inventions. The uncertainties lie not in knowing what to do, not in science, and not in economics. The uncertainties lie in our ability to discipline our individual and collective wills to act with courage and compassion. A health care system as efficient and fair as it is miraculous is at last within our reach, if we have the daring and persistence to finish the health care revolution.

TRENDS IN THE HOSPITAL SECTOR

Peter D. Kralovec, BA
Director, Hospital Data Center
American Hospital Association
Chicago, IL

The initial goal of this paper was to describe the hospital sector of the health care delivery system. Since, however, the industry contains 7,000 institutions that employed 3.6 million people and generated over $100 billion in expenses in 1986, a detailed presentation is obviously impossible in the limited space available. Accordingly, I will restrict my discussion to certain important general trends.

ADMISSIONS

According to the AHA's National Hospital Panel Survey, the recent falloff of inpatient admissions first began in 1983, when admissions fell slightly (by 0.5 percent). Sharp drops (around 4 percent) followed in 1984 and 1985. Year-end data for 1986 indicate that the admission decline moderated to 2.1 percent. Variations among bed-size groups were significant, however, ranging from a 13.5 percent decline among hospitals with fewer than 25 beds to a 0.2 percent increase in those with 300 to 399 beds.

LENGTH OF STAY

For the first time since 1981, average length of stay increased, rising to 6.6 days. The increase was consistent in the under-65 and over-65 age groups. Its occurrence in the face of incentives for shorter stays suggests a rise in the severity of illness among inpatients, as more of the less severely ill patients are treated on an outpatient basis.

11

INPATIENT DAYS

Inpatient days fell by 1.4 percent in 1986—not a sharp decline when compared with those in 1984 (8.9 percent) and 1985 (6.2 percent). Since 1981, inpatient days have fallen by 18 percent, with 50 million fewer patient days in 1986 than in 1985, while outpatient visits have risen by 19 percent. With respect to bed size, a fairly consistent pattern is evident: the smaller the hospital, the larger the decline. Declines in inpatient days between 1981 and 1986 ranged from 43.5 percent among hospitals with fewer than 25 beds to 9.7 percent among hospitals with more than 500 beds. In part, this reflects a long-term trend toward fewer hospitals in the smaller bed-size categories and more in the medium to large bed-size categories. According to AHA analysis, of the 71 community hospitals that closed in 1986, more than three fourths had fewer than 100 beds, even though only half of all hospitals fall into that size category. Between 1975 and 1985, the number of community hospitals with fewer than 25 beds fell by 30 percent.

OUTPATIENT VISITS

In recent years, health care providers have successfully shifted the emphasis in health care practice from inpatient care to ambulatory care. Technologic advances in diagnostic imaging, surgery, and anesthesiology have combined with changes in reimbursement policy and provider practice to fuel strong outpatient growth, which resulted in 263.6 million visits in 1986. Outpatient visits rose by 4.8 percent and 8.3 percent in 1985 and 1986, respectively, after several years of relatively modest growth.

DIVERSIFICATION ACTIVITIES

In addition to performing more ambulatory surgical activity, hospitals are diversifying into nonsurgical outpatient care. Between 1981 and 1985, the number of community hospital-based outpatient departments rose by 27 percent, the number of alcoholism and chemical dependency outpatient programs rose by 30 percent, the number of outpatient rehabilitation programs rose by 17 percent, and the number of outpatient psychiatric programs rose by 11 percent. Moreover, hospitals are becoming more involved in sponsoring freestanding ambulatory care centers. Health promotion and home health care have also been big growth areas. More than half of all community hospitals offered health promotion programs in 1985, whereas only 40 percent did in 1983. Furthermore, almost 1,600 community hospitals, or 30 percent, reported offering home health care services in 1985, whereas only 15 percent did two years earlier.

INFLATIONARY PRESSURES

Inflationary pressures—as measured by the AHA market basket index based on a sampling of products and services used by hospitals—eased for hospitals in 1986, slowing from a 5.9 percent rate in 1985 to a 5 percent rate. Nonlabor inflation slowed more abruptly than labor inflation. A lag in hospital inflation, particularly for wages, is not surprising. After a shift in general economic inflation, it normally takes up to 18 months before that change is incorporated into hospital purchasing and wage contracts.

Despite the slowdown in labor inflation, it appears likely that hospitals will continue to face upward pressure on labor costs from factors unrelated to general economic inflation, such as shortages of workers in particular job classifications and a shift toward higher occupational skill mixes. For example, a recent analysis in Monitrend, a report by the AHA's Hospital Administrative Services, shows a shift toward greater use of registered nurses in medical and surgical units and less use of nonprofessional staff. Several reasons may account for this shift: administrators may be restructuring staffs to improve labor productivity, or else more acutely ill inpatients may require more care from higher skilled workers.

PERSONNEL

One of the side effects of greater outpatient volume and slower inpatient day declines has been a turnaround in the decline in utilization of full-time equivalents (FTEs). Employment of FTEs increased by 0.3 percent, after declining by more than 2 percent in 1984 and 1985. According to AHA field surveyors, individual hospitals report difficulty in matching staff increases in their outpatient service areas with staff reductions in inpatient areas, because more severely ill inpatients require more intense labor utilization. Nonetheless, since 1983, hospitals have employed approximately 133,376 fewer FTEs.

As for bed-size variations, hospitals in half of the eight bed-size groups continued to experience FTE declines, mainly in the smallest and largest bed-size categories. Those bed-size groups that exhibited FTE increases also had above-average outpatient visit growth, below-average inpatient admissions declines (or admissions increases), or both. The growth rate for part-time employees was greater in 1986 (0.9 percent) than that for full-time employees (0.2 percent). The percentage of total personnel who are full-time employees has fallen steadily over the past decade, from 77 percent to 72 percent.

Demand for registered nurses, both within and outside of hospitals, remains strong. According to the AHA's Annual Survey of Hospitals, the total number of registered nurse FTEs on community hospital payrolls increased by

1.6 percent overall between 1983 and 1985. During this same time period, total FTEs decreased. The percentage of FTEs accounted for by registered nurses in community hospitals increased from 22 to 23 percent. Concurrently, the number of licensed practical nurse FTEs dropped by 18.7 percent, and the decline in the number of FTEs in all other categories averaged more than 3 percent. Between 1980 and 1984, the number of nurses employed by hospitals rose by 21 percent. In 1985, hospitals employed 789,000 RNs. Growth in nurse employment in ambulatory care settings, including physicians' and dentists' offices, health maintenance organizations (HMOs), and ambultory care centers, and in the public and community health sector was even faster: 35 percent and 22 percent, respectively. These trends reflect not only rapid growth in ambulatory and home health care opportunities, but also the potentially greater attraction of some aspects of nonhospital employment for nurses, such as greater flexibility in choice of hours and less evening and weekend work. These data, then, may suggest that hospitals will face increased competition for nurses' services from other types of employment settings.

STAFFED BEDS

For the third successive year, the number of staffed beds declined. Staffed beds peaked in 1983, at 1,004,000; since then, they have declined by more than 40,000. The decline in staffed beds and a more moderate inpatient day drop have combined to stabilize occupancy rates. Occupancy rates averaged 63.4 percent in both 1985 and 1986, after three years in which occupancy rates fell by an averge of 3.6 percent each year.

REVENUES

In the past three years, the patient revenue growth rate has lagged markedly behind the rates of previous years. The inpatient revenue growth rate has lagged even further behind. The outpatient revenue growth rate, which has remained strong over the decade, slowed from 18.7 percent in 1985 to 17.3 percent in 1986, despite a sharp upswing in outpatient volume.

EXPENSES

The total expense growth rate was higher in 1986 (8.9 percent) than in 1985 (6.6 percent). The acceleration was driven by more rapid nonlabor expense growth—fueled in part by outpatient service expansion—and an overall increase in FTEs, stemming from slower inpatient day declines and faster outpatient visit growth. The 1986 expense growth rate, however, remained below the 14.8 percent average annual rate for 1977 through 1983.

The labor expense growth rate also accelerated, but more moderately, increasing from 5 percent in 1985 to 7.3 percent. In contrast, labor expenses per FTE actually slowed from 7.4 percent to 6.9 percent.

REVENUE MARGINS

Revenue margins dipped sharply in 1986, as revenue growth lagged behind expense growth. Net patient margin dropped by more than half, from 1.5 percent in 1985 to 0.7 percent in 1986, while total net margin fell from 6 percent to 5.1 percent. Revenue margins have been falling since 1984.

UTILIZATION TRENDS

Despite a sharp decline in revenue margins, 1986 data suggest that many hospitals are in fact preparing for future demands. Reports from field surveyors suggest that the acceleration in expense growth in 1986 stems in large part from increased costs related to outpatient service expansion. Although hospitals continue to face inpatient day declines, the decline was moderate in 1986, compared with 1984 and 1985. Continued cost containment activities among other payors will probably continue to bring declines in inpatient days, but those declines may be less dramatic than in the past. The sharp growth in outpatient activity in 1986 indicates that hospitals are successfully shifting the emphasis of health care practice toward ambulatory care. As more care is diverted to outpatient settings, the patients remaining in acute care beds will be more severely ill, which exerts upward pressure on length of stay. The extent to which this increasing pressure on length of stay can be offset will be governed in part by the availability of alternative levels of care. The number of skilled nursing beds, long-term care facilities, and home care programs, in turn, will be influenced by reimbursement policies for those settings.

FUTURE EXPENSE GROWTH

It is difficult to predict the future pace of total expense growth. The lower general inflation rate in 1986 will probably begin to affect hospitals more strongly in 1987, bringing a moderating influence. If a large portion of the acceleration in 1986 can be attributed to the expansion of outpatient services, and that expansion reflects new business ventures, then expense growth is likely to moderate in 1987. New ventures require significant startup costs, and productivity levels normally do not peak until six months to a year after startup. According to a 1986 AHA survey of ambulatory care, however, 78 percent of 2,200 hospitals surveyed intend to expand their ambulatory services. If a large proportion of those hospitals have yet to complete those projects, expense growth may continue to face upward pressure.

Hospitals face at least two other obstacles that could adversely affect expense growth, both in 1987 and in the long run. Malpractice insurance costs continue to rise sharply, despite efforts in some states to curtail them. Sharp rises here have a noticeable impact on total expense growth. Furthermore, recent reports of a nursing shortage could place hospitals in a poor position to bargain for lower wage increases.

OUR NATIONAL POLICY: MATERNAL-CHILD HEALTH

Marianne Roncoli, PhD, RN
Assistant Professor
University of Pennsylvania
Philadelphia

Karen Gallo, RN
Level III Practitioner
Hospital of the University of Pennsylvania
Philadelphia

Health policy is a decision backed by the authority of government that determines who in the population receives services; what services will be delivered; and where, when and how these services will be distributed. The success of this policy depends upon the extent to which health care goals are realized. Sidel and Sidel (1977) suggest goals that a responsible society might have for its health care system, including creating a fair and equitable distribution of health services; strengthening individual, family, and community life; protecting health; and caring for the ill and the "worried well."

How successful have our health policies been in achieving these goals? Although the right to vote and the right to an education are not questioned in our society, the right to health is still not considered a prerogative of citizenship. A just, fair, and equal distribution of health service has eluded us; we seem only to be struggling to reduce inequities in health care delivery. We wish to strengthen individual family and community life, but many of our health care programs provide episodic, disruptive care that disregards the family. In many instances, the current trend toward home care instead of expensive hospital care in order to contain costs denies the hidden cost to families—especially to women, who assume the burden of caring for themselves, their children, and their aging parents in the home without adequate support services.

We wish to protect health, yet few services are made available for and few dollars spent on primary, preventative health care. We care for the ill very well, but we lack a comprehensive, supportive approach to care preferring instead to emphasize emergency care and expensive hospital procedures.

How successfully have we met these goals especially as regards maternal-child health (MCH)? The answer depends on a review of who receives services, what services are delivered, and when and how they are delivered.

WHO RECEIVES MATERNAL-CHILD SERVICES?

The recipients of maternal-child health care are pregnant women and their children. From 1969 through 1975, 86 percent of all women received prenatal care, 72 percent in the first trimester (Pratt, 1982); however, the Institute of Medicine reports that the improved use of prenatal services, especially during the first trimester, is decreasing, particularly for women under 15 years of age (*Preventing Low Birth Weight,* 1985). Most recently, 5.7 percent of all women receive no prenatal care. For all black women and black women under 15, the figures were 9.9 and 19 percent, respectively (Marieskind, 1980). Gains that were achieved have been lost. For all the efforts being made, health care is not reaching poor women, especially poor women from minority groups. Black children, for example, are twice as likely to die in the first year of life, be born premature, suffer low-birth-weight, and have mothers who receive no prenatal care, and three times as likely to be poor, have their mothers die in childbirth, be mentally retarded, die of child abuse, and be in foster care, than white children are. Of all births to black women, 58 percent were out of wedlock. In black women under the age of 20, 86 percent were out of wedlock (Edelman, 1987).

Although U.S. women live an average of 75 years, in 1975 they were ranked ninth in the world in longevity, behind the women of Norway, Sweden, the Netherlands, France, Canada, Japan, Denmark, and Switzerland (Marieskind, 1980). In infant mortality, a country's leading indicator of maternal-child health, the U.S. is still 15th in the world; in 1982, U.S. infant mortality was 11.2/1,000 live births (Roemer, 1986). The U.S. maternal mortality of 11.2/100,000 live births—7.7/100,000 for white women and 26/100,000 for minorities—is also higher than that of 11 other industrialized countries (Marieskind, 1980).

Most babies are still born to women 20 to 24 years of age, and half are born to women who work during their pregnancy (Marieskind, 1980). Also, one-fifth of all births to women aged 15 to 44 are not wanted at the time of conception. Before the 1973 Supreme Court decision legalizing abortions, 329 women were reported to die from abortion each year; only 15 died after abortion-related procedures in 1977. However, about 30 percent of women who wanted abortions could not get them. Medicaid-eligible women have an abortion rate three times higher than that of middle- or working-class women (Lewin & Olesan, 1985).

Many of the women who seek maternal-child health services are poor. In 1984, four out of five families receiving Aid to Families with Dependent Children (AFDC) were headed by women. Of all AFDC recipients, 68 percent are children, and half of these are eight years old or younger; 45 percent are eligible because their parents are divorced or separated. In 1984, one in nine children in America were dependent on AFDC, and one in four children will depend on AFDC at some point in their childhood (Edelman, 1987).

Those who receive services, then, are likely to be women of early child-bearing age, either sick or disadvantaged with limited resources, and working to provide those resources. Their children share their disadvantaged position.

WHAT MATERNAL-CHILD SERVICES ARE BEING RECEIVED?

When service delivery is examined, the limitations of our health policy emerge. Some government agencies provide direct service, most finance health care, and some others regulate it (Roemer, 1986). In the executive branch of government (see Table 1), the State Department contains the Agency for International Development, which provides technical assistance to developing countries in the areas of nutrition, family planning, environmental health, and MCH. The Department of Agriculture is responsible for the national school breakfast and lunch programs, food stamp programs, and the Women,

Table 1.   U.S. Government Agencies Involved in Maternal-Child Health

State Department
Department of Agriculture
Department of Defense
Veterans Administration
Health and Human Services
   Human Development Services
   Health Care Financing Administration
      Medicare (Title XVIII)
      Medicaid (Title XIV)
   Social Security Administration
      AFDC (Title IV, Title V)
   Public Health Service
      Center for Disease Control
      Food and Drug Administration
      Health Resources Administration
      Health Services Administration
      National Institutes of Health
      Alcohol, Drug Abuse, and
         Mental Health Administration

Infants, and Children (WIC) Program. The Department of Defense operates medical and health care programs for the armed services. The Veterans Administration operates the largest system of public hospitals and clinics in the country.

The Department of Health and Human Services administers the majority of programs. The Office of Human Development Services, through the Administration of Children, Youth, and Families, directs the Head Start Program and Programs to Combat Child Abuse and Neglect. It gives developmental disabilities program grants to states, offers special projects funding, and supports university-affiliated centers for handicapped children and a vocational rehabilitation program providing funds for testing, guidance, training, and placement of handicapped youngsters, as well as living services (Wallace & Medina, 1985).

The Health Care Finance Administration assumes the enormous task of financing health care for the poor and the elderly. Approximately 40 percent of health care in America is financed by the federal government (Roemer, 1986). The two major programs are Medicare and Medicaid. Medicaid, or Title XIX of the Social Security Act, makes provision for the indigent, those receiving public assistance, those receiving AFDC, and those who are medically indigent. A large part of this program pays for the health care of mothers and children. It is funded in part by the federal government and in part by the state that administers the program. The Social Security Administration provides welfare to mothers and children at the state level as well. Established by the Social Security Act of 1935, Aid to Dependent Children (ADC) preserved elements of the original legislation that established widows' pensions. In 1950, Congress added a caretaker grant to provide for the mother's essential expenses and changed the name of the program to AFDC (Sidel, 1986).

Another source of federal support administered by the state is Title V, which allows block grants for MCH and crippled children services. Title V contains two funds. Fund A provides for MCH services at the state level in accordance with the number of live births; this allotment is matched by the states. Fund B is unmatched, and the amounts it provides are dependent on states' financial need. Half of Fund B is used by the Federal Office of Maternal-Child Health for special regional grants or projects, such as maternal-infant care (MIC) projects, dental health, family planning, and intensive care for newborns. According to the provision of Title V, each state must provide a project in each of these categories.

The U.S. Public Health Service administers many programs that affect women and children, including the Centers for Disease Control and the Food and Drug Administration. The Health Resources Administration includes the Bureau of Health Manpower, of which the Division of Nursing was a part. The Health Services Administration manages the Office of MCH, family planning, migrant health, community health centers, rural health, and the National Health Service Corps. The National Institutes of Health, of which the Center for Nursing Research is now a part, encompasses many institutes, including the National Institute of Child Health and Human Development (Wallace & Medina, 1985). Finally, the legislative branch of the federal government has committees that decide health-related matters (see Table 2) (*Congress and Health,* 1985).

This review of services highlights the fragmentary nature of maternal-child health service delivery. On the whole, the government finances health care rather than provides the actual service itself. The government acts as a third-party payor for the practitioner in private practice. It is largely in the business of insurance rather than of health care delivery.

WHEN AND HOW ARE SERVICES DELIVERED?

Maternal-child health services are primarily delivered when women and/or children are acutely ill or pregnant. In 1980, 40.3 percent of all health care expenditures went for in-hospital care, 18.9 percent for ambulatory and in-patient care by physicians, and only 3 percent for public health services (Roemer, 1986). In 1930, there was one primary care provider for each 1,000 people; in 1970 there was one provider for every 2,000 people (Roemer, 1986). These figures suggest that primary health care—including health screening and promotion, which are vital to the protection of the health of pregnant women and children—is not well financed. Obviously, the goal of protecting health cannot be met, given the above expenditures. The Institute of Medicine, in its 1985 report on preventing low birth weight, has outlined a program for the delivery of prenatal services that is designed to enroll women during

Table 2. U.S. Congressional Committees Addressing Health Care Issues

Senate Committees

    Labor and Human Resources
    Agriculture
    Finance
    Select Committee for Indian Affairs
    Armed Services
    Environment and Public Works

House Committees

    Energy and Commerce
    Agriculture and Nutrition
    Ways and Means
    Armed Services
    Education and Labor

the first trimester. The report recommends that additional funding for Medicaid and the MCH block grants be provided and that states and local governments design services for high-risk women that address *all* the barriers to prenatal care, whether in the health care delivery system, in the providers, or in the patients themselves. Care should be culturally and ethnically sensitive, personalized, and accessible to transportation and that makes provisions for child care. A public relations campaign should be formed, the report continues, to reach the community, where pregnant and potentially pregnant women can learn of the importance of prenatal care and nutrition, the dangers of substance abuse, and the need for a stress-free environment. The Healthy Mothers, Healthy Babies Coalition, a four-year-old consortium of over 80 national voluntary, professional, and government organizations, including the American Nurses' Association, the Nurses' Association of the American College of Obstetrics and Gynecology, and the National Association of Pediatric Nurses Associates and Practitioners, is asked to coordinate community efforts (*Preventing Low Birth Weight,* 1985). A prenatal program has been outlined.

Maternal-child health services are delivered episodically. They are designed to deal with situational and developmental crises—pregnancy, child birth, illness—not to provide comprehensive care. Only ten states provide comprehensive services; five states do not reimburse clinic services, and nine do not reimburse nurse midwives. Even given adequate reimbursement, many physicians do not accept Medicaid, and the reimbursement provided is well below what the physician charges (Gold & Kenny, 1985).

Nowhere is the lack of comprehensive service more dramatically illustrated than in the care of low-birth-weight infants. Although Medicaid will provide reimbursement of over $20,000, on average, and sometimes as much as $1,000,000 for the care of a low-birth-weight infant in the hospital (Roncoli & Brooten, 1986), little money is made available for comprehensive follow-up. Even though the use of a clinical nurse specialist for home follow-up following early discharge has been demonstrated to result in a cost saving of $18,000 per infant, this program is not widely implemented by hospitals. It is a relatively expensive program to run. A hospital administrator would prefer to keep the baby longer in the hospital, where reimbursement for intensive care charges is guaranteed, rather than pay clinical specialists for follow-up services that are reimbursed at a rate of about $15 per home visit.

Maternal-child health services are inequitably delivered under the control of the states rather than of the federal government. Despite a 1961 reform that permitted states to extend aid to families with dependent children that had an unemployed father in the home, only 26 states have elected to use this option. A child in Mississippi in 1983 received $0.99 per day, or $30 per month; Alaska, on the other hand, provided $5.96 per day. In contrast, SSI provided $7.59 per day or $231 per month for a disabled individual. This differential can be attributed to how funds are distributed. The state sets AFDC limits, while the federal government sets limits for SSI (Sidel, 1986).

Does AFDC really help families climb out of poverty? A report by the Children's Defense Fund suggests that it does not: the payments are just too low. There have been two major cutbacks in this program, one in 1981 and another in 1983. Also, new provisions were included, such as lowering the eligibility level and changing the calculation of income; counting a step-parent's income, regardless of whether the income is available to the child; and not allowing federal AFDC assistance to women pregnant with their first child until the sixth month of pregnancy, while at the same time increasing the waiting time for assistance. Moreover, since 1981 the states have had the option of including the value of food stamps and housing subsidies in deter-mining eligibility and benefit level, along with the option of allowing recipients to "work off" the value of AFDC grants, usually by doing manual, unskilled, badly paid, difficult work (Edelman, 1987).

At best, these provisions are an embarrassment to a humane and decent government; at worst, they are motivated by mean-spirited, selfish legislators and policy makers. These provisions only make the poor poorer; they are a punishment for being poor. Furthermore, if a woman is pregnant, the above provisions actually make it harder for her to gain access to prenatal health care. Since the benefits do not become available until well into the second trimester, she may delay seeking prenatal care. She probably will not be able to afford to travel to a health care site frequently. Since her food allotment will be included within her AFDC payment, she will probably receive inade-quate nutrition. Furthermore, having to work off her AFDC payment will create additional stress, which is exacerbated by worry about how to makes ends meet with less available. With respect to the IOM report on preventing low birth weight, it is clear that these AFDC regulations will foster rather than prevent the birth of a low-birth-weight infant.

Restriction on the distribution of MCH services is nowhere more evident than in the practice of abortion. Since the passage of the Hyde Amendment in 1977, which restricts the use of federal Medicaid funds for abortion to cases in which the life of the mother is in jeopardy, the abortion option for poor women has been impossible or very difficult to exercise. One fifth of all U.S. countries have no abortion providers. However, Lewin and Olesan (1985) report that more than 90 percent of Medicaid women who seek abor-tions can get them, though at great personal and family expense.

Maternal-child health services, then, are distributed inequitably by the states, primarily when women and children are sick. The care is primarily episodic, and it is available only when a person becomes poor—or very poor. It is also restrictive in that it punishes women for getting pregnant without adequate means, rather than makes the means available.

CURRENT LEGISLATIVE REFORM

As regards the goal of equal access to MCH services for all, certain legislative reforms present hopeful signs that we can still "tinker" with the health care system in such a way as to generate a coherent, comprehensive health policy. The 1987 Medicaid Infant Mortality Amendment (*Congressional Record,* 1987) of the 1986 Omnibus Reconciliation Act allows states to expand Medicaid eligibility to 186 percent of the federal poverty threshold ($16,165 for a family of three); it also mandates that states cover all children aged five to eight whose family's income is below the state poverty level. Introduced by Senator Bill Bradley of New Jersey and Representative Henry Waxman of California, this legislation, if passed, will provide more financing for MCH care. Even if it is passed, however, it remains to be seen how the states distribute the funds. Perhaps, all MCH services provisions should, like Social Security, be determined by the federal government. It is no surprise that those countries with better infant mortality and morbidity statistics than our own have made a societal commitment to assume responsibility for the health and welfare of children through government-supported MCH services that are easily accessible and usually free.

Besides additional appropriations or MCH (Title V) block grants being considered by the 100th Congress, legislation to mandate family and medical leaves of absence from employment has been proposed in both houses of Congress. This legislation provides for up to 18 weeks of maternity leave and up to 26 weeks medical leave for both men and women (Foye, 1987). If enacted, these bills will encourage the development of family life, a major health care goal. It is important, however, to remember that this legislation will *regulate* business practices to foster family health; it will not provide additional service, nor will it finance health care.

The 99th Congress established the National Commission to Prevent Infant Mortality. Designed to study MCH services in a comprehensive fashion nationwide, this commission should make the country aware of the inadequacy of our current MCH policy; however, it too will neither finance care nor provide service. Until policy makers go beyond studying and regulating, the system of care delivery will not change. If health care goals in America are to be realized, the government must mandate what the citizenry will not provide. We cannot afford to take a *laissez-faire* approach to health care.

In the meantime, we can support legislative reform, while remaining alert to those reforms that harm women and children. Professional nurses can join and support the professional societies and private sector associations that attempt to influence legislation on MCH on the local, state, and national levels, such as Perinatal Associations, the Children's Defense Fund, and the March of Dimes. Finally, self-help efforts such as the LaLeche League and the Black Women's Health Project should be supported. Coalitions between the private and public sector, however flawed, are the best way of mandating a national comprehensive MCH policy that will enable health care goals to be met.

REFERENCES

Brooten, D., Kumar, S., Brown, L., Butts, P., Finkler, S. A., Bakewell-Sachs, S., Gibbons, A., and Delivoria-Papadopoulos, M., et al. (1986).

A randomized clinical trial of early discharge and home follow-up of low birth weight infants. *New England Journal of Medicine, 315,* 934–939.

Congress and Health (16th ed.) (1985). New York: National Health Council.

Congressional Record, Proceedings and Debates of the 100th Congress, First Session, *133*(14), January 29, 1987.

Edelman, M. W. (1987). *Families in peril: An agenda for social change.* Cambridge: Harvard University Press.

Foye, G. J. (1987). Family and medical leave act of 1987—HR 925/5.249. *Bulletin: National Perinatal Association, 2*(2), 10.

Gold, R. B., & Kenny, A. M. (1985). Paying for maternity care. *Family Planning Perspectives 17*(3), 103–111.

Lewin, E., & Olesan, V. (Eds.) (1985). *Women, health, and healing: Toward a new perspective.* New York: Tavistock Publications.

Marieskind, H. I. (1980). *Women in the health system.* St. Louis: C. V. Mosby, Co.

Pratt, M. W. The demography of maternal and child health. (1982). In H. M. Wallace, E. M. Gold, & A. C. Oglesby (Eds.), *Maternal and child health practices: Problems, resources, and methods of delivery.* New York: John Wiley and Sons.

Preventing Low Birth Weight. (1985). Division of Health Promotion and Disease Prevention, Institute of Medicine. Washington, D.C.: National League Academy Press.

Roemer, M. I. (1986). *An introduction to the health care system* (2nd ed.). New York: Springer.

Roncoli, M., & Brooten, D. (1985). Caring for low-birth-weight babies. *Nursing and Health Care 6*(4), 198–201.

Sidel, R. (1986). *Women and children last.* New York: Viking.

Sidel, V. & Sidel, R. (1977). *A healthy state.* New York: Pantheon.

Wallace, H. M., & Medina, A. S. (1985). The organization of a legislative base for health services for mothers and children. In M. M. Wallace, E. M. Gold, & A. C. Oglesby (Eds.), *Maternal and child health practices: Problems, resources and methods of delivery.* New York: John Wiley and Sons.

EDUCATION

AN UPDATE ON THE NATIONAL COMMISSION ON NURSING IMPLEMENTATION PROJECT: EDUCATION

Colleen Conway-Welch, PhD, CNM, FAAN
Professor and Dean
Vanderbilt University School of Nursing
Nashville, TN

The National Commission on Nursing Implementation Project has defined the role of its workgroups as essentially that of "think tanks." These think tanks collect and review published and unpublished data that identify nurses' agreement on the issues facing nursing and the significance of current and future trends in health care. Then, using nurses' agreement as a base, the workgroups design action strategies. We workgroup members structure our discussions and activities in ways that allow us to meet our yearly objectives and to send the results of our deliberations to the Governing Board. The Governing Board then goes through a consensus-building process focusing on the workgroup reports and recommended strategies. It identifies actions on which all members of the Board can agree and sends the results of its deliberations out to the public, primarily via its own organization.

It is important to emphasize that what the three workgroups send to the Governing Board is raw data; thus, there are and will be differences between what the Governing Board receives and the finished product it sends out. Consequently, we in the workgroups have a mandate to present to the Governing Board what we collect as the mainstream of thought on an issue; we influence the role of the Governing Board through the information we collect, review, and present to them. The Governing Board then takes our work and determines where and how the various organizations can take action.

YEAR 1

During year 1, the Workgroup on Nursing Education (Workgroup I) addressed the following objective: Nursing must outline a common body of

29

knowledge and skill essential for basic nursing practice, the curriculum content that supports it, and the credentialing process that reinforces it. The activities involved in year 1 included the following:

1. A review of published and unpublished data on future projections of health care consumer needs, nursing service needs, and nursing education needs,
2. A review of these projections with a view to providing a data base and a rationale for change in nursing education, and
3. A projected timeline for change in nursing education, which has as a goal the preservation of all money from federal, state, local, and private sources that are presently being spent on nursing education.

The results achieved during year 1 are as follows:

1. A document was drafted describing the future of nursing and the health care delivery system as we see it. The Governing Board received that document and is restructuring it into a document unique to their vision of the future.
2. A second document was drafted that had to do with the characteristics of the professional nurse and the characteristics of the technical nurse. This was sent to the Governing Board and was accepted by them.
3. A timeline for change, entitled "Timeline for Transition Into The Future Nursing Education System for Two Categories of Nurse," was drafted. The draft was sent to the Governing Board and was accepted by them.

These results were achieved by focusing on (1) describing the characteristics of nurses needed in the health care delivery system in the year 2000 and (2) identifying the type of change needed in nursing education programs to ensure an adequate supply of appropriately prepared nurses in the year 2000. The supply issue was of great concern to the work groups as well as to the Governing Board. We know as a profession that our present efforts are not maintaining even the current supply of nurses, let alone an adequate supply. We know that change is vital if we are even to maintain our current supply, which is still insufficient.

The development of the timeline was one of the most exciting activities that occurred in year 1. It is present-oriented, in that we are using it to represent many changes that have already started to occur, and also future-oriented, in that we know that all programs will change, because we will need different practitioners in the year 2000. Even the current associate degree and bachelor of social nursing programs will have to change in order to prepare people to work in the future health care delivery system. This timeline recognizes that this change has already started and suggests how we can manage change and address the shortage issue in a proactive, positive manner.

Nursing has not managed change well in the past. We have a way of holding onto both the successes and the problems that are a part of our history. But nursing today is different. All the data available to the workgroups suggests that nursing is now eager to manage change successfully. *Manage* is a key word for our future.

YEAR 2

Having completed the work of year 1, the Workgroup on Nursing Education moved to the year 2 objective: describe curriculum models for nursing programs that are in transition from one type of nursing program to another, and set forth those models that provide excellence in education and promote development of effective practitioners capable of responding to the future needs of clients. The activities involved in Year 2 included the following:

1. Developing a questionnaire that was sent out to programs to create a checklist of inhibiting and facilitating factors that a program needs to consider when initiating change; and

2. Inviting Dr. Cele Lenagacher, Director of the Associate Degree Program at Manatee Junior College in Florida, to present her American Hospital Association–commissioned study of models of change developed by diploma schools that have made transitions.

The results achieved already during year 2 are as follows:

1. The second national invitational conference will be held in November to discuss the results of year 2.

2. A questionnaire was developed by staff that incorporated all major categories that needed to be managed when programs are changing from one to another. It was found that a major inhibiting factor to program change was our own nursing colleagues and that a major facilitating factor was the chair or dean of the program and the faculty. These findings will be made available to programs considering change or in the process of change. We believe that they can assist programs during the change process.

3. We acknowledged that the diversity of our current and future students is increasing, that a large share of future nursing students will be adult learners, and that the teaching-learning process used in nursing education must incorporate new teaching strategies and new learning strategies to attract and keep students.

4. Programs must be offered in the most productive, cost-effective, and cost-efficient methods possible.

These results were achieved by focusing on (1) describing educational models that currently exist and that are undergoing change, (2) describing inhibiting and facilitating factors that influence the success of those programs,

(3) addressing issues related to the teaching-learning process within the context of the timeline developed in year 1, (4) exploring ways in which we can supply socialization in nursing that allows nurses to change according to the timeline, and (5) realizing that ultimately all current nursing programs must change in order to produce the new technical nurses and professional nurses needed by the year 2000.

We planned the last meeting of Workgroup I before the National Invitational Conference so that we could continue to review the impact of the timeline on these programs.

We are all looking forward to the Second Invitational Conference as a means of further communicating the results of our efforts and to further our goals as an implementation project. Change has already begun to be implemented in nursing education, and we want to assist it in every way possible.

ENTRY-LEVEL GRADUATE EDUCATION IN NURSING: MASTER OF SCIENCE PROGRAMS

Barbara D. Schraeder, PhD, MSN
Associate Professor
Rutgers University/Camden
New Jersey

In 1983, Slavinsky, Diers, and Dixon wrote a prize-winning article describing a new trend: the increasing numbers of college graduates seeking entry into nursing programs. They estimated that this group constituted 5 percent of the nursing population. They also listed a variety of entry options available to this mature, well-educated group: diploma, associate degree, baccalaureate degree, masters degree, and doctorate. Four years later, this "hidden" group, as it was called, is becoming an increasing focus of interest, for a number of reasons.

- The end of the baby boom generation has eroded the numbers of 18–20 year olds who have traditionally entered nursing programs and enrollment is declining, forcing programs to find new markets for recruitment.

- Changes brought by DRGs with mandated specialized care, coupled with the explosion in technology and the concomitant social and ethical problems that are now entangled with health care, support the need for better educated, more sophisticated nurses.

- There is an increasing number of learned and thoughtful nurses who agree with Luther Christman's (1987) statement that there is a social mandate for health care practice that is beyond the baccalaureate level. It is no longer appropriate or excusable for nurses to be among the least educated members of the health care team. It is a waste of talent and ability to direct college graduates into programs offering less than graduate education.

There are two programs that can be entered at the graduate level: the nursing doctorate (ND) program and the master of science degree program. Both programs specifically build on the educational strengths and life experiences of non-nurse college graduates who seek professional education in nursing. They do not rework a college degree; rather, they use it as a foundation. This paper describes the six programs offering graduate education at the master's level to non-nurse college graduates.

THE PROGRAMS AND THEIR CORE BELIEFS

All six programs were surveyed: Massachusetts General Hospital Institute of Health Professions (MGHIHP), Pace University, the University of Tennessee in Knoxville, Vanderbilt University, Yale University, and McGill University. The programs all reflect the belief that a completed undergraduate education with all that it engenders, is the foundation for professional education in nursing. There is the assumption that an individual entering a nursing program should already possess the intellectual characteristics of an educated person at the time of entry. Several leaders who were surveyed cited the American Associations of Colleges of Nursing's document "Essentials of College and University Education for Professional Nursing" (1986) as expressing their beliefs about the foundations for professional education. The essential characteristics noted in the document include the abilities to write and speak effectively, to think critically, to use a second language, to understand mathematical concepts and the physical world, to appreciate art, to comprehend the meaning of human spirituality, and to make ethical judgments in both personal and professional life. The leaders' beliefs about the effects of a liberal educational foundation reflect Derek Bok's (1986) idea that "a critical mind, free of dogma, but nourished by human values, may be the most important product of education in a changing fragmented society" (p. 47). Like Bok, they also believe in the value of an educational experience that includes a wide range of extracurricular activities and life experiences.

The second core belief of five of the programs (those of the MGHIHP, Pace, the University of Tennessee in Knoxville, Vanderbilt, and Yale) is that graduate education in nursing implies specialization. There is a pragmatic as well as a philosophical base for this belief. Some leaders decried the "ambiguity" inherent in a generalist degree and pointed out that there is no such thing as a generalist practice. All of us are called upon to work in specialized settings, even those who work as staff nurses in general hospitals. Another reason for offering a specialty Master's degree is the perceived need for a program that imparts clearly defined marketable skills to individuals who will have a minimum of six years of higher education at the completion of the nursing program. The exception to this view is McGill University, which has resisted the temptation to specialize and provides a generalist experience which stresses critical thinking, broad-based principles that transcend settings, and the application of research skills and principles to the practice of nursing.

PROGRAM CHARACTERISTICS

All but one of the programs, that in the University of Tennessee at Knoxville, are in private universities. All either have a tradition of graduate specialty education or (in the case of the MGHIHP), offer only graduate degrees.

The programs differ on prerequisites. Some, such as those of Yale and the MGHIHP, have none, admitting individuals with a variety of undergraduate degrees—e.g., music, art, psychology, and English majors—as well as those with science backgrounds. These programs tend to place an emphasis on life experiences, looking for individuals who are committed to learning and who possess critical thinking and study skills. The other programs are more traditional in their approach to prerequisites, requiring students to possess credits in anatomy, physiology, chemistry, and microbiology. The programs without prerequisites report that their students do well without them. They have developed, as part of the professional education curriculum, graduate level science courses that are relevant to the science of nursing. Yale, for instance, has a course entitled "Biomedical Sciences" and the MGHIHP has one called "Biophysical Sciences."

All of the programs are intense and range from two to three years in length. The first four to six semesters have been labeled the "bridge," the "generalist," or the "basic" curriculum, depending on the institution. At the end of the bridge (to use Vanderbilt University's term), three of the schools provide recognition that that phase of the educational experience has been completed. Pace confers a bachelor of social nursing (BSN) degree, whereas Yale and the MGHIHP give a certificate. At Pace, the MGHIHP, and Yale, students may sit for state boards upon completion of the BSN or the certificate portion of the program. The reasons for this tend to be pragmatic as well as philosophical. Acquiring a license to practice confirms students' identities as nurses; it also, enables them to work part-time as registered nurses. At that point, students begin their specialty education. All of the programs offer a wide menu of specialty options, and this may be an important part of their success in attracting students. Class sizes range from 20 to 50 students.

All schools clearly articulated the aspects of the students' experience that characterize their programs as graduate education. There is a wide use of seminar learning experiences, and research is emphasized in all aspects of the curriculum. The case study methodology is often employed. The educational experience is a fully collegial one, with a great deal of discussion and dialogue, which encourages assimilation and accommodation of learning to world experiences and previous education. The students are not viewed as tabulae rasae, their professional education builds on their unique strengths.

STUDENT CHARACTERISTICS

The students' average age is 28 to 29 years, with a range of 22 to 50. Two of the program directors noted that the average age is drawing closer to that of the typical college graduate, for many students appear to be electing to enter professional nursing education during their senior year in college or after a short experience in the work world. The students have been described as bright, well-educated, and possessing a "heightened sense of dedication to human kind." They are also characterized as very sharp and able to articulate well-formulated political and social views. The percentage of men in the group appears to be slightly higher than the norm (5 to 10 percent).

The directors identified three major groups of college graduates who seek graduate education in nursing. The first group comprises individuals who late in the college experience identified nursing as a career interest and who recognize the lack of extrinsic value in a baccalaureate degree in our society. These individuals specifically want a graduate degree. The second group is made up of the "people" types. These are individuals who have been active in altruistic occupations or avocations and who now seek a degree that gives them flexibility and the skills to do important "people-oriented" work. Many of these students have had Peace Corps experiences, belong to the clergy or religious, or have been active in the consumer health movement, (for instance, in La Maze, Women's Health, the Cancer Society, or the like). The third group has been labeled "mysterious." These are the individuals who have had no apparent previous health care interest. Some may have had an ill parent or relative and been impressed by the nurses who provided care. Others may have done volunteer work and found themselves suddenly attracted to a caring profession. Still others may simply have been unhappy with their previous job. They may have been bored, not advancing quickly enough, or induced by some internal force to change careers.

Non-nurse college graduates choose graduate programs in nursing for a variety of reasons.

- They see the extrinsic value of a graduate degree and come specifically for that.

- Graduate specialty education provides a confirmation of a life interest in a particular specialty.

- They want to move ahead in their careers and perceive a second baccalaureate degree as a step backwards.

- They want to be part of a growing profession, and they are responding to the many advertisements for nurses that fill the newspapers each week.

- They have a strong commitment to patient care and they believe that these programs will give them the skills to practice well.

The commitment to practice is reflected in the choices the students make after graduation. Many go immediately into specialty practice. They become certified in their specialty and assume these roles. Others need time to confirm their abilities and seek traditional entry-level positions. Many graduates move into entrepreneurial roles and leadership positions.

CHALLENGES

Three challenges were identified by the leaders of five of the programs: marketing, faculty resources, and cost. The older schools report relying on word of mouth to publicize their programs. In recent years, they have had to step up their efforts to attract applicants. The new programs, such as Vanderbilt, have started out with very sophisticated and beautiful brochures and creative marketing strategies. Most of the schools draw from a national student body. A marketing strategy that holds promise is the use of the popular press. One school reported that seven applications resulted from an article in *Glamour* magazine. *Working Woman's* recent description of nursing as both one of the 20 worst careers and one of the 25 best has an impact on these innovative programs. The areas of nursing growth identified in the article are clearly the bailiwick of the well-educated, creative students these programs expect to attract—that is, the corporate nurse, the wellness nurse, and the nurse consultant. The popular press has been identified as a great help, but it is also a great hindrance, especially in those articles that focus on poor pay, poor working conditions, and powerlessness in nursing.

A positive image in the national press and in the national communication network was identified as a key variable in attracting college graduates into nursing. All of the programs have increased their marketing budgets and have developed strategies for tapping into the college-educated market. Some schools have targeted the Peace Corps, Vista, and religious communities as likely sources of applicants. A particularly effective marketing device has been the senior year at Vanderbilt program. Vanderbilt University has initiated contracts with a variety of undergraduate institutions to provide their students with the senior year bridge. After the bridge year, students return to their respective colleges, graduate, then come back to Vanderbilt University for their specialty education. This program has generated 11,000 inquiries.

The second challenge is finding and retaining the right mix of faculty. The faculty must reflect the competence in research and scholarship that one would expect in a graduate faculty, have a commitment to and expertise in specialty practice, and be comfortable in a collegially based educational experience for adult learners. The non-nurse college graduate students of nursing were described as challenging and continually questioning. Their considerable repertoire of positive life experiences has fostered self-confidence, intellectual curiosity, and self-direction. It takes an open, highly competent, self-assured faculty with a well-developed sense of humor to establish a supportive milieu.

Accompanying the challenge of finding the right mix of faculty is that of finding the educational resources. Since most generalist nursing education takes place at the undergraduate level, most texts are directed at that level of student. Some schools describe a heavy investment of faculty time in developing their own learning materials.

Cost is the third challenge. With a 1/5 faculty/student ratio, these programs can be expensive. Students, especially in those programs without prerequisites, have highly individualized learning needs and goals. Attracting and retaining doctorally prepared faculty and those with expertise in a clinical specialty often requires schools to meet the salaries common in private industry. Thus, the costs of faculty and educational resources may be quite high.

The programs are costly for students as well. All require a full-time commitment. The students at the generalist, or bridge, level are often ineligible for the traineeships and stipends that traditionally fund graduate education. The ability to work as a nurse after the generalist foundation is an attraction for students in some programs, but there is a need for continuous and creative searching for funds for students.

If one wishes to identify two overarching ideas that have emerged from this survey, two words come to mind: commitment and creativity—commitment to a vision of education based on a sound philosophical base and pragmatic facts and creativity in program development and in the meeting of challenges. Professional graduate education for non-nurse college graduates is no longer a curious phenomenon; it is an important trend.

REFERENCES

American Association of Colleges of Nursing. (1986). *Essentials of College and University Education for Professional Nursing: Final Report.* Washington, DC: Author.

Beyers, M. (1987). Future of nursing care delivery. *Nursing Administration Quarterly, 11*(2), 71–80.

Bok, D. (1986). *Higher education.* Cambridge: Harvard University Press.

Christman, L. (1987). The future of the nursing profession. *Nursing Administration Quarterly, 11*(2), 1–8.

Forni, D. (1987). Nursings' diverse master's programs: The state of the art. *Nursing and Health Care. 8*(2), 71–75.

Graduate program in the biological, agricultural, and health sciences (21st ed.). (1987). Princeton, NJ: Petersen's Guides.

Hechinger, G. (1987, April). Nursing careers: New and improved. *Glamour,* p. 344.

Konrad, W. (1986, July). The 25 hottest careers of 1986. *Working Woman,* pp. 65–73.

Slavinsky, A., Diers, D., & Dixon, J. (1983). College graduates: The hidden nursing population. *Nursing and Health Care, 4*(7), 373–378.

Smith, R. (1976). Why college graduates in nursing. *Nursing Outlook, 24*(2), 88–91.

ACKNOWLEDGMENTS

The author wishes to thank Dr. Beth Grady, Dr. Veronica O'Day, Dr. Mildred Finsky, Dr. Colleen Conway-Welch, Judith Krauss, MSN, Dr. Laurie Gottlieb, and Amy Harshman for their time and good humor in sharing facts and ideas about the programs.

THE PROFESSIONAL DOCTORATE
AS AN ENTRY LEVEL INTO PRACTICE

Jean Watson, PhD, RN, FAAN
University of Colorado Health Sciences Center
Denver

In discussing the important topic of postbaccalaureate doctoral education for nursing's future, I prefer to sidestep the issue of "entry into practice" and focus instead on the profession's role and responsibility for health care in society. Once the appropriate and necessary curriculum is developed to prepare nurses as full health professionals with the essential liberal education and clinical base, then academic institutions will grant the degree that is merited by the nature of the program and the professional outcomes. Thus, the degree that is granted is secondary to the discussion. I submit, however, that the appropriate and necessary postbaccalaureate curriculum for nursing's future will merit the professional nursing doctorate, the ND degree.

Such a bold initiative for nursing's future is proposed as a national model at the University of Colorado School of Nursing. The program plans to build upon the experience of Case Western Reserve University and expand the concept of the ND degree by introducing an autonomous health and human caring professional nursing program. The program would incorporate advanced practitioner skills (physical as well as psychosocial), while also introducing a new curriculum focusing on human caring, health, and healing that links humanities and science, thereby more fully actualizing the art and science of nursing.

SUPPORT SYSTEMS

The systematic support systems in place to establish the Colorado model in health and human caring, include the following:

- A local network of national and international advisory boards and community leaders;

- Establishment of the new Center for Human Caring as the focal point for experimentation with curriculum, new practice roles, teaching-learning methods, and interdisciplinary links;
- Supported by the infrastructure of the Center for Human Caring for academic and clinical practice programs through faculty and resource development and clinical agency collaboration;
- Formal policy analysis of the program in society and health care delivery systems through special projects with the University of Colorado Center for Ethics and Health Policy in Denver;
- Links with clinical agencies to introduce and demonstrate new roles and functions for the ND graduate in traditional and nontraditional health care agencies;
- An approved third-party reimbursement process through new 1987 state legislation in Colorado;
- Use of national networks such as the American Association of Colleges of Nursing (AACN) for dissemination of the model curricula and program to other university schools of nursing and health sciences center campuses; and
- Experimenting with and evaluating innovative, collaborative, and autonomous practice roles for advanced nurse clinicians, while simultaneously developing the model academic program.

The structure and support system for developing and implementing a postbaccalaureate health and human caring program is critical, because it has to be supported by faculty, colleagues, and society. Changes such as these are underpinned by several additional rationales. For example, six significant reports published in the past five years regarding the quality of education in the United States (Sakalys & Watson, 1985) support postbaccalaureate professional education and better links between science and the humanities. In general, all major study recommendations include the following (Sakalys & Watson, 1985, p. 298):

1. Restoration of the centrality of the liberal arts in professional education;
2. Increased curricular structure and coherence;
3. Increased emphasis on intellectual skills, such as analytic, problem-solving, and critical-thinking skills;
4. Increased emphasis on mastery of basic principles rather than specific facts;
5. Increased emphasis on fundamental attitudes and values;
6. Increased emphasis on lifelong learning;
7. Decreased specialization at the undergraduate level; and
8. Increased emphasis on broad and rigorous baccalaureate education prior to professional education.

In addition to curriculum reform, the studies also make the following administrative recommendations (Sakalys & Watson, 1985, p. 299):

1. Increased leadership and support for educational reform and rigor;
2. Revision of reward structures to promote high-quality teaching;
3. Faculty development to promote good teaching and the acquisition of new forms of instruction; and
4. Increased support for educational research.

Such prominent studies and consistent recommendations support the need for nursing to reexamine the adequacy of current levels of preparation. In particular, increasing concern regarding the excessively vocational and narrow nature of professional education and the erosion of liberal education is leading to a restructuring of all professional education, including baccalaureate nursing education. In response to such concerns, it is incumbent on nursing to reflect seriously on its activities in curriculum development, instruction, and administration. The reports' recommendations can lead the way.

NURSING CURRICULUM

The postbaccalaureate nursing curriculum at the University of Colorado, which is based upon the national studies, can emphasize the interplay between humanities and biomedical science by means of the following:

- A more extensive liberal arts foundation, coupled with better understanding of an appreciation for cultural diversity and the human, subjective dimensions of health–illness experiences;
- Critical thinking and advanced problem solving, contributing to clinical judgments and independent decision making;
- A core knowledge underpinning of biomedical science, social behavioral science, and organization-system management theory and practice;
- More extensive philosophical ethical decision-making skills based upon ethics of human caring, which attends to the contextual, relational, emotional, "behind the scenes" ethical dilemmas (which are often invisible), as well as the traditional rationalistic approach to biomedical ethics;
- More value-laden theory associated with human caring transactions, emphasizing self-care and more autonomous decision-making processes as important client goals in health care; and
- A human caring theory-based nursing curriculum, including the latest research on and knowledge of human caring practices and systems of caring, emphasizing the relationship between human and system caring approaches and health–healing outcomes, regardless of medical diagnosis and treatment regimens.

The practice skills of the postbaccalaureate graduates will include the following:

- Traditional nursing skills and techniques, along with advanced practitioner skills of both a primary and a tertiary nature, including physical and psychosocial assessment and management skills, especially in relation to gerontology clients, chronically ill clients, children and adolescents—all within the context of human caring values, ethics, and knowledge;

- New human caring practice modalities that incorporate natural healing modalities (along with traditional medical treatment regimens) and the role of aesthetics in caring e.g., use of music and human movement, in conjunction with other health-healing approaches that complement and balance traditional medical approaches, such as stress management, therapeutic touch, imagery, therapeutic massage, advanced interpersonal communication, and health teaching–learning skills; and

- Options in supportive-elective coursework and clinical practice, along with experiences in areas such as administrative management, clinical education, and focused clinical areas of practice (e.g., acute-progressive life threatening illness, or health-wellness self-care).

In addition, the new graduates will be able to initiate clinical nursing research as well as participate in such research. Baccalaureate graduates do not have sufficient research skills to design and implement clinical research projects independently. During the model program, students will conduct clinical research studies.

In general, the new postbaccalaureate graduate will have a background in the art and science of human caring and will be skilled in a wide variety of caring and health-healing modalities. Such nurses will demonstrate an appropriate balance between "high tech" and "high touch" in their practice. Baccalaureate programs do not provide the time necessary to build a sufficient background in both the biomedical and the human caring dimension; therefore, nurses from traditional programs are more oriented to the biomedical and technological aspects of nursing and are not prepared to function as full professionals (Tate, 1987).

NEW ROLES AND CHANGES
IN THE HEALTH CARE SYSTEM

Because of future changes projected for health care, the envisioned model program graduate (Watson, 1987) will discard the non-nursing functions, tasks, and responsibilities that can be performed efficiently by others and will function as a scholar-clinician. Crucial human caring knowledge and practices considered to be the best of current nursing practice will be retained and expanded (A. Smith, personal communication, 1987). In addition, the new graduate will assume some responsibilities and roles previously in the realm of medicine or other domains. Thus, the postbaccalaureate graduate will be prepared as an autonomous full health professional, one who is capable of making independent and critical clinical judgments. The ND will function as an advanced nurse clinician, in and out of institutions, homes, clinics, and alternative care settings. The practitioner will be able to follow individuals and groups of patients on a continuous care basis in and out of hospitals and other systems, and will directly provide, oversee, and coordinate continuous caring for groups of people in a society and health care system that is rapidly changing.

The health care delivery system of the future is envisioned as a multifaceted, complex system of choices, in both traditional and nontraditional settings. Hospitals will continue to decline and will accommodate only the most severely and acutely ill. Home care, family-oriented care, and self-care will continue to grow as persons become more informed about, responsible for, and assertive on behalf of their own health care needs. The role of a full health professional nurse in and out of institutions—i.e., to deliver expert caring and provide, oversee, and coordinate advanced health-healing practices—will be a critical and continuing role in society. Indeed, some futurists suggest that expert caring nurses as health professionals will be the only continuous care providers in the future in a largely depersonalized, technologically oriented, fragmented system of care.

Eventually, the model program will merit the ND and allow the nurse (prepared as the caring specialist in the system) to function as a full health professional. This will help to bring about a new social order in the traditional health care delivery system and will open up new continuous care options for health care in society. The proposed ND will fill a void in the traditional medical-dominated illness-focused system.

SUMMARY

Although nursing entered the academic environment over 70 years ago, its educational practices for preparing professionals have yet to incorporate the full professional academic model. Professional nurses are still educated at the baccalaureate level, with minimal preprofessional general education requirements. A convergence of social, educational, and professional trends, however, clearly indicates a need for a professional nurse with a different type of preparation.

Given nursing education's current structure and the needs of the future, nurse leaders and major schools of nursing have the responsibility to take a philosophical position regarding professional education and thereby fashion appropriate curricula for the year 2000. Accordingly, the School of Nursing faculty at the University of Colorado Health Sciences Center believes that the preferred future is a postbaccalaureate educational program meriting the ND. The rationale for this position is consistent with the 1828 Yale report, the Flexner and Goldmark reports, and the 1984–1985 reports on higher education in the United States, as well as with the University's and the School's role and mission in the state.

The University of Colorado faculty's rationale can be summarized as follows: (Sakalys and Watson, 1986, pp. 91–97). The faculty believes that nursing is a rapidly growing human science that focuses on the human care aspects of health care delivery at both the individual and the system level across the lifespan. Such a belief acknowledges that the separate paths of sciences and humanities are converging in light of resurgent interest in the human caring dimensions of health and illness and increasing recognition that complex problems in health and illness are inherently multidimensional.

Two principal outcomes are expected at the University of Colorado:

- In the short term, a national model for postbaccalaureate professional nursing education that is consistent with recent trends in higher education and emphasizes liberal arts and social sciences as necessary foundations for professional education; and

- in the long term, the development of a cadre of health professional nurses for the 21st century who are prepared to deal creatively, coherently, and humanely with the ethical, technical, and scientific issues and values that are emerging as critical elements in nursing and health care practices.

Our challenge now is to create a preferred future in which nursing merits the status of a scholarly discipline that can actualize both its epistemic and its social mission. It is not a matter of the doctorate as entry into practice, but a matter of the doctorate as the degree merited (in a restructured postbaccalaureate curriculum) if nursing is not only to survive, but also to follow the necessary educational and clinical requirements mandated by transformations in the health care system of today and tomorrow.

REFERENCES

Flexner, A. (1960). *The Flexner report on medical education in the United States and Canada 1910.* Washington, DC: Science & Health Publications. (Reprinted from Carnegie Foundation for the Advancement of Teaching, 1910, Bulletin Number Four, New York: Author).

Goldmark, J. and the Commission for the Study of Nursing Education. (1923). *Nursing and nursing education in the United States.* New York: MacMillan.

Hofstadter, R., & Smith, W. (1961). *American higher education: A documentary history, Volume I.* Chicago, IL: University of Chicago Press.

Sakalys, J., & Watson, J. (1985). New directions in higher education: A review of trends. *Journal of Professional Nursing, 1,* 293-299.

Sakalys, J., & Watson, J. (1986). Professional education: Post-baccalaureate education for professional nursing. *Journal of Professional Nursing, 2,* 91-97.

Tate, J. (1986-1987). *ND task group documents.* Denver: University of Colorado School of Nursing.

Watson, J. (1979). *Nursing: The philosophy and science of caring.* Boston: Little, Brown and Company. (Reprinted by the Colorado Associated University Press, Boulder, Colorado, 1985).

Watson, J. (1987). *A humanitarian-based caring curriculum.* Unpublished manuscript prepared for Kellogg Foundation.

Watson, J. (1987). *A national model of postbaccalaureate nursing education.* Unpublished manuscript prepared for Kellogg Foundation.

THE PROFESSIONAL DOCTORATE
AS AN ENTRY LEVEL INTO PRACTICE

Michael A. Carter, DNSc, RN
University of Tennessee, Memphis

This paper is built on two assumptions: first, that preparation for the professional practice of nursing must rest on a liberal undergraduate education, and second, that professional educational programs that prepare the practitioner in the art and science of nursing must lead to the professional doctorate, the ND. These critical assumptions are the logical derivation of an assessment of the current health care system, the ever-expanding nursing science base needed for professional practice, and the projected evolution of the practice of nursing in the years ahead. These two assumptions are interrelated but will be discussed separately.

REQUIREMENT OF A LIBERAL EDUCATION BEFORE ENTRY INTO THE PROFESSIONAL NURSING PROGRAM

Nursing is a peculiar discipline. The central focus of nursing is the care of humans by themselves and by others. Human care occurs during all stages and phases of development and in virtually all settings in which humans exist. This central focus of human care requires an understanding and commitment to a world view of humans as indivisible whole beings embedded within a co-extensive context. In juxtaposition to nursing's focus upon holistic human caring phenomena, other health disciplines focus on parts of the whole or on particular curative tasks aimed at parts. This dialectic of whole and parts means that the professional practitioner of nursing must form a synthesis of these two points of view in order to assist the recipient of care in making some logical, rational sense of an extremely confusing system. Not only must the professional nurse be highly competent in the provision of human care, he or she must also be exceedingly knowledgeable about other health professions.

What, then, is the body of knowledge needed to form the basis of practice? In other words, what are the basic fields of study for nursing practice? This question can best be answered by returning to the central focus of nursing practice. Basic to understanding human care are those areas of study that are uniquely human. These include the unique human biology, the formation of human relationships, the formation and development of language, and the expression of the human condition through the arts. The basic fields of study for the aspiring nursing student include both those that are particularistic, such as psychology, sociology, anthropology, and biology, and those that are not, such as languages, music, art, and history (American Association of Colleges of Nursing [AACN], 1986).

The next question to be asked is, What are the ways of thinking needed for the professional practice of nursing? Again, the central focus of nursing provides some clues. Nurses must understand human values and ethics, moral judgments, political systems, religion, and spirituality, as well as mathematics and philosophy (AACN, 1986). The blending of the basic fields of study with the multiplicity of ways of thinking forms the minimum base on which professional nursing education should be built. To understand people and the context in which people exist, nurses must have this broad base of knowledge and ways of thinking. I agree with Sakalys and Watson (1986) that this broad base cannot be learned without a number of years of college-level study. To do less severely limits the practitioner and, more important, does not provide for fully competent professional practice.

Built on this broad base of liberal education, the professional program prepares practitioners of nursing to fully execute their abilities at the conjunction of the human arts and science. The professional program based on a liberal education enhances the practitioner's abilities to understand, to think, and to care in ways not possible under our current system of nurse education. The evidence is clear and compelling.

Professional practice education cannot be adequate if the practitioner is ignorant of the development and expression of the contributory arts and sciences, their inherent richness, and their limits for human care. Even to think that a professional nurse can be prepared without at least a baccalaureate-level liberal arts preprofessional education is to live in a delusional world. There is no other professional practice that focuses on whole people in synergistic evolution with their context. The body of knowledge and ways of thinking required for professional practice are more complex in nursing than in any other health profession.

We are hindered in fully appreciating this, however, by the very nature of the practice of nursing. Nursing practice can appear to be deceptively simplistic. Much of nursing practice is assisting the person in meeting basic human needs. Even the name we use for our field, "nursing," indicates a basic biologic phenomenon of mammals. Yet the full meaning of the concept of nursing is so subtly and profoundly rich that its depth is usually understood only by those who have been the recipient of high-level nursing care or by those who spend substantial time in study of the discipline.

WHY THE PROFESSIONAL DOCTORATE
FOR NURSING PRACTICE?

To understand our system of health care delivery, we must attempt to understand the insidious and widespread influences of sexism. Throughout the last century, the positions of power and authority in health care were held by an elite few. These power elites were able to overthrow all of the competing ideologies and medical theories to ensure the rise and success of allopathic medicine. All other views were seen as not being formed in the likeness of science and therefore as being either religious beliefs or superstitions. The study of allopathic medicine was (and continues to be) viewed as the most important form of study in the health sciences. Fields such as dentistry and pharmacy were allowed to grow primarily because they were male-dominated and were considered a subset of allopathic medical practice. Other fields have not fared so well.

Nursing has always run a double risk. First, the practitioners have been almost exclusively female. This means their work, like most women's work, is seen as being of significantly less value than men's work. This problem has been further compounded by the denial to men of access to nursing education and positions of influence in nursing. Nursing has been designed to remain women's work. Second, the world view of nursing, which does not give primary importance to reductionistic, Western science, is viewed by power elites as being flawed and insufficient. The movement of the locus of education of nurses from hospitals to colleges and universities did not help as much as might have been expected. Perhaps this is because a substantial portion of the practice of nursing continues to take place in elite-dominated and highly authoritarian settings, such as the hospital.

As we examine the professional practitioners in the U.S. health care system, we note an interesting finding: the one field that has the most all-encompassing practice has the lowest level of educational attainment. In pharmacy, medicine, and dentistry, practitioners begin their professional practice at the doctoral level, and other fields, such as occupational therapy, physical therapy, and social work, are rapidly moving to master's- and doctoral-level entry. A skeptical response would be that if nursing were considered men's work rather than women's work, the issues surrounding doctoral-level entry would have been resolved over a century ago.

My point is that to be full members of the cadre of health care practitioners, professional nurses of the future must hold equivalent degrees. The programs of study must be as rigorous as or more rigorous than those of the other disciplines. To do less harms the public we purport to serve.

This harm results from two sources. First, without holding credentials equivalent to those of other health care professionals, nurses continue to be devalued as less educated, regardless of the facts of the situation. For this reason, I believe that entry at the master's level in nursing, as is the case in a number of schools, does not alter the power relationships in the necessary fashion and does not advance the profession. Professional nurses must be doctors, as pharmacists, dentists, and physicians are. Without being doctors, nurses cannot adequately hold their own in the advancement of health care for their clients vis-a-vis other providers.

The second source of harm, and perhaps the more damaging, is the inability to control the knowledge base for the discipline. The art of the discipline is the creative exploitation of the science of nursing for the betterment of human care. The practitioner who enters the field at the doctoral level is expected to make a very different use of the science base in practice than is the practitioner with less than doctoral preparation (Fitzpatrick, Boyle, & Anderson, 1986). The doctoral level nurse practitioner demands that the knowledge be structured to allow understanding of whole persons within their context. Particularistic sciences are viewed by the doctoral-level nurse practitioner as interesting but limited. Without entry at the doctoral level, nurses are not able to exercise these prerogatives.

My point of view is that programs that prepare nurses for entry into professional practice in the future must be at the postbaccalaureate level and must culminate in the professional doctorate, the ND. To do less will mortally wound the practitioner and will deny the public the full potential of professional nursing practice.

REFERENCES

American Association of Colleges of Nursing. (1986). *Essentials of college and university education for professional nursing.* Washington, DC: Author.

Fitzpatrick, J. J., Boyle, K. K., & Anderson, R. (1986). Evaluation of the doctor of nursing (ND) program: Preliminary findings. *Journal of Professional Nursing, 2,* 365–372.

Sakalys, J. A., & Watson, J. (1986). Professional education: Postbaccalaureate education for professional nursing. *Journal of Professional Nursing, 2,* 91–97.

THE PROFESSIONAL DOCTORATE
AS AN ENTRY LEVEL INTO CLINICAL PRACTICE

Joyce J. Fitzpatrick, PhD, RN
Professor and Dean, Frances Payne Bolton School of Nursing
Case Western Reserve University
Cleveland, OH

The strong demand for registered nurses generally is augmented by an even stronger demand for nurses prepared at advanced levels. Presently, a small minority of professional nurses are prepared at the master's and doctoral levels. We have a shortage of leaders in nursing and a great demand for nursing leadership. The doctor of nursing (ND) program is designed to address this leadership need.

BACKGROUND

Early in the 1970s, the faculty of the Frances Payne Bolton School of Nursing, under the visionary leadership of Rozella Schlotfeldt, began discussions and deliberations about a professional doctorate as the entry-level educational preparation for professional nursing. The idea for such a program was indeed revolutionary at the time of its introduction. In 1972, only seven doctoral programs in nursing existed: three offering the PhD or research doctorate, three offering clinical doctorates for advanced specialty practice (the DNS or DNSc), and one offering the EdD. The idea of doctoral education *within* nursing was a novel one, as was the idea of doctoral preparation *for* nurses. In the early 1970s, fewer than 500 nurses with any kind of doctoral preparation could be identified. Additionally, the great debate regarding basic levels of nursing education, which is still present in our profession, was paramount at that time.

In May 1978, the classic pioneering article by Schlotfeldt, entitled "The Professional Doctorate: Rationale and Characteristics," appeared in *Nursing Outlook*.

On the basis of an analysis of the needs of the health care delivery system, the status of nursing as an academic discipline and an autonomous profession, and the existing cadre of nursing practitioners, Schlotfeldt argued that the time was right for introducing the professional doctorate as a desired educational option for entry into professional nursing practice.

Several aspects of Schlotfeldt's original presentation are worthy of note here. First, the basic argument proposed was that of nursing's scientific responsibility to focus on a holistic understanding of human health. The conceptualization of nursing as a scientific discipline was of primary significance in developing the program. Second, Schlotfeldt was concerned with aspects of implementation of the professional nursing role, including issues of collaborative health care practice, status issues, and the strongly identified need to advance both nursing education and professional nursing practice. Third, Schlotfeldt further explicated characteristics of the students, the faculty, the locus of study, and the curriculum and its organization that were perceived as essential program dimensions. The first ND students were admitted to the program and began their three-year course of study in the fall of 1979. In May 1982, 34 persons grduated from the ND program. At present, there are approximately 200 ND graduates. Six classes have graduated, and we have just admitted our ninth class.

FACULTY PHILOSOPHY

We faculty members believe that nursing is both an academic discipline and a profession. As an academic discipline, nursing is a distinctive branch of human knowledge fundamental to nursing practice, education, and administration, and to the continuous development of the profession. The distinctive perspective of nursing is that which defines the domain of professional nurses as the multiple dimensions of human health. The body of nursing knowledge is continuously advanced, structured, and restructured through scientific research and inquiry and dynamic interplay between professional nursing practice and research. As a profession, nursing involves assisting persons in the maintenance of health, detecting deviations from health, assisting persons in the restoration of health, and supporting persons during life. These responsibilities are accomplished through a systematic and deliberative process, a process that requires strong collaboration among health professionals and between health professionals and the public.

Through the ND program, we prepare nurses to initiate a range of opportunities for their professional practice. Further, we provide individuals with the knowledge, skills, and values for clinical practice, clinical scholarship, and for a professional career. As a clinically competent practitioner of nursing, the graduate is expected to be proficient in professional nursing skills; to engage in autonomous, collaborative health care practice; to display interpersonal competence; to assume a leadership role in nursing; to demonstrate the ability to manage health systems and resources; and to practice at an advanced level in a selected area. As a clinical scholar, the graduate is expected to use theoretical and empirical knowledge; to know and apply the process of theoretical thinking; to use and test concepts, models, and theories; to use and explicate the rationale and data for clinical nursing decisions; to critically analyze nursing phenomena and evaluate clinical situations; and to systematically study a selected area in order to advance practice in that area. As a professional, the graduate is expected to be ethical in decision making, to display professional values, and to assume responsibility for his or her own learning and professional growth. As a health care professional, the graduate is expected to understand the management of information and systems, to analyze systems to implement change, and to influence health policy and planning. The ND program is characterized by educational depth and an emphasis on inquiry and collaboration in patient care, which are also hallmarks of other health professions. It is our belief that the strong undergraduate educational preparation that the student brings, plus the comprehensive professional and clinical course of study of nursing offered through the ND program, will enable nurses to function effectively as partners with other professionals in the provision of quality health care.

ND CURRICULUM

The ND program of study is three academic years, for a total of six semesters. Year 1 focuses on basic nursing knowledge and skills, emphasizing the development of a nursing perspective and knowledge about human health. Students explore the practical and theoretical frameworks that form the bases for practice. Learning experiences in year 2 include the extension of clinical experience and the use of nursing interventions with persons in various patient populations. Students participate in beginning courses on nursing theory and nursing research with other beginning graduate (MSN) students in the School of Nursing and with students in other professions (law, medicine, social work) in a multidisciplinary course in professional ethics.

Year 3 focuses on development of knowledge and skills for advanced clinical nursing practice. This year includes an opportunity for students to select a focal area for concentrated clinical practice. Students extend their emphasis on clinical inquiry through two concentrated nursing research seminars. They choose an area for inquiry and participate in a clincial evaluation project that will be formally presented as a major project of the professional education. As this component of the program continues to be strengthened, it is expected that through these clinical studies students and faculty will make a major contribution to the clinical nursing literature and to clinical nursing practice. For example, it is our expectation that ND students and faculty will choose to publish their clinical studies in the new journal *Applied Nursing Research,* soon to be launched by the faculty of the

Frances Payne Bolton School of Nursing. During Year 3, the student is also introduced to important material on health policy and planning and information systems and management.

Through completion of the curriculum, the student achieves a professional doctorate and receives a preparation for professional nursing practice that is truly comparable to the traditional professional preparation of physicians, dentists, and lawyers. It is our plan to make opportunities for expanding their education available to ND students in the summers following years 2 and 3. Clinical options for specialization and career options, such as teaching, administration, and health care management, will be available.

FUTURE FOR ND GRADUATES

Perhaps the most frequent questions asked are, What do your graduates do? and Where do they practice? As a result of a three-year project funded by The Cleveland Foundation, we have some beginning data regarding the ND graduates from the first three classes, i.e., those who graduated in 1982, 1983, and 1984. Generally, the study results indicate a strong professional career commitment among ND graduates, who consistently describe themselves as leaders and as professionals. The majority of graduates assumed clinical practice positions immediately after graduation and stated that their need for attaining additional clinical experience was one of the primary motivating factors in selecting these first positions. Many graduates reported strong and continued interest in advancing their education through continuing education, clinical specialization, or more in-depth research. Employment flexibility and mobility were evident among these early program graduates; both lateral and hierarchical position changes were recorded. Further, ND graduates expressed a desire to explore nontraditional practice settings and nursing practice roles.

I continue to be enthusiastic about the future potentials for the discipline of nursing, particularly as I interact with the women and men who are choosing the ND program as a way of actualizing their commitment to humankind. We have now developed the professional security and confidence among a core group of nurse leaders that will allow us to transmit our continued commitment to caring for people in all phases of health and illness, in a variety of clinical settings, so that we may all experience a better quality of life and health. We can accomplish our goals through the ND program.

REFERENCE

Schlotfeldt, R. M. (1978). The professional doctorate: Rationale and characteristics. *Nursing Outlook, 26*(5), 302–311.

CURRICULUM: RESTRUCTURING FOR PRACTICE

Lucille A. Joel, EdD
Chairperson, Department of Adults and the Aged
Director, Teaching Nursing Home Project
Rutgers University College of Nursing
Newark, NJ

The purpose of this paper is to present my views on the inadequacies of education for entry into nursing practice and to propose curriculum changes that I believe would enhance the position of nursing practice in the 1980s. I will intentionally avoid debating what educational credentials are appropriate for the registered nurse. It is enough to say that we are faced with an evolving health care system that demands artful and intelligent nursing practitioners, and that the brightest and the best will be attracted to nursing only if the field promises status and rewards.

The success of any educational program is measured against its ability to attract students and to produce a product that is relevant and valued in the workplace. The world of work for both nurses and individuals who are making occupational decisions has changed dramatically over the past years. One could conjecture that many of our current nursing shortage problems can be traced to the fact that nursing has not remained sensitive to the desires of those who are making career decisions or to the demands of the marketplace. Nursing has become less appealing as a field of work, yet more nurses than ever are needed. This situation, however, should be considered from the perspective that all shortages are self-limiting: they either correct themselves or are corrected by social readjustments. Society created the physician's assistant in times of physician undersupply and the licensed practical nurse as a response to the nurse shortage of past decades.

ATTRACTING STUDENTS
FOR CONTEMPORARY NURSING PRACTICE

The future of any educational program depends on its ability to attract students. People currently choosing an occupation are making decisions on the basis of their personal needs and are less ready than they once were to pursue a career for purely altruistic reasons. Altruism was once a popular motive for selecting a career in nursing. In recent studies, however, young people who are making initial occupational choices report that financial compensation is highly important to them. They are not ashamed of their materialism or of their desire to achieve status and personal expression in their work (Green, 1987). They report, in fact, that status and pride in work are even more important than financial compensation. According to some studies, salary increases have to be in excess of 15 percent to serve as an important incentive (Pinchot, 1985). The recruitment picture for nursing is further complicated by the appeal that the field holds for students who are transferring from other areas of study, second-degree students, and older adults making a career shift. This situation merits careful investigation, along with program design and marketing tailored to attract diversified audiences.

The health care delivery system is unsettled and often hostile. Health care providers are jockeying for survival. Social workers are taking over discharge planning and case coordination. Health educators intrude on the comprehensive care that characterizes nursing. Physicians are trying to recapture the clinical management prerogatives they relinquished during periods of shortage. These are examples of the multiple turf battles which exist. Providers who survive and thrive will become established on the basis of cost-efficiency and therapeutic outcomes. Historical patterns of blind trust between the provider and the recipient of care are being replaced by consumer demand for accountability based on objective criteria. For nursing, the subjectivity of caring must be translated into demonstrable benefits.

Service settings and the nature of services are equally unsettled. In an attempt to cut costs, health care resources are being directed away from acute care facilities and toward alternate settings for care that promise to be more economical (Joel, 1985). Home health care and community-based services have experienced unprecedented growth in recent years (American Nurses' Association, September 1984). Predictions indicate an eventual reduction of more than 30 percent in acute care beds. Conversely, fully maintaining the sick or the frail in the community may exceed the cost of institutional care. The standards for the service delivery setting and the nature of service still remain unclear.

The health market, though largely unreimbursable, is burgeoning. Unfortunately, nursing has been associated with medicine, illness, and hospitals in the minds of the consumer. In fact, 65 percent of nurses are still employed in hospitals (American Nurses' Association, 1985). The economic assault on hospitals and the fact that nurses are the single largest manpower group in this labor-intensive industry targeted nursing for cutbacks. Nursing positions vacated by attrition were left unfilled, and salaries were frozen. Aides and licensed practical nurses were substituted for registered nurses in an effort to cut costs (Joel, 1987). More recently, the clinical demands on hospitals, in terms of sicker patients and increased technology, have created a demand for registered nurses and in many instances have led to improved salaries. Demand exceeds availability, however, which results in a poor work environment for hospital nursing. ("The Debate," 1987).

A health care environment that has been honestly described as unsettled and to some degree hostile demands nurses who are assertive, strong in their practice, and steadfast in their convictions. Pioneers of this sort are necessary to salvage deteriorating and eroding markets for nursing and to develop new markets. Personality testing to preselect or counsel students in their occupational choices may be in the best interests of both the profession and the individual.

Much of nursing's current inability to capture more power and prestige is a direct result of our reluctance to accept expanded responsibility and our distaste for assertive action and unpleasantness. It should be noted that nurses still have an exceptionally positive image with the consumer. In a recent public opinion survey, consumers saw nurses as the group that could most logically help curtail health care costs by expanding their usual activities. Consumers thought that nurses should be able to perform physical examinations and prescribe medications (American Nurses' Association [ANA], July 1985). It seems that the only people who have reservations about nurses are nurses themselves. Today, when professionals in all categories have lost much of the respect they were once accorded by society, nurses have maintained a good image. We should take steps to capitalize on that situation immediately; as anyone who scans the press regularly knows, we may soon lose this consumer edge. Articles in magazines and newspapers not uncommonly attribute hospital fatalities and inadequate health care to the absence of seasoned and experienced nurses ("New York Hospital on the Spot," 1987). Reports like these will begin to chip away at the good reputation of the profession. It remains to be seen whether nurses, if they become more assertive and politically astute, can fare better.

There are indications that some of our recruitment woes would be alleviated by increased direct public funding for nursing students and professionals recruitment of students. The ranks of nursing swelled when the nurse cadet corps was formed during World War II. Several colleges of nursing have achieved a dramatic increase in applications by investing in public relations and sophisticated recruitment programs. But attracting students is not enough: only timely and relevant nursing education will enable them to enrich and be enriched by practice once they graduate.

PRESCRIPTION FOR CURRICULUM CHANGE

Given the "information age" we live in, it is difficult to avoid a content-laden curriculum. Academic medicine and academic law have compensated by using process as content. Beyond the basic level, content is given a case orientation and used as an instrument for developing process skills. The art of medical and legal education is to cultivate a professional approach to problem identification and resolution. Beyond accepting process as content, a highly conceptual curriculum can allow the graduate to better accommodate to rapid change in any scientific field.

It becomes difficult to reconcile these educational principles with an employment setting that expects a confident practitioner. The gap between the conceptual and the concrete has to be bridged by case method, simulations of clinical management, and computer-assisted instruction. This gap is particularly wide and deep in regard to bioinstrumentation and medical devices. Educational programs have commonly minimized any obligation to develop technologic competence in their graduates. Many nurses never rise above their initital discomfort with devices and instruments and become controlled by technology. These circumstances have given rise to new disciplines such as bioengineering, and a host of technicians. The problems with practice encroachment follow closely behind. These problems will grow as technology leaves intensive care and finds its way onto the acute care unit and into the nursing home and the community. A relevant curriculum for the 1980s must include a heavy dose of physics, equipment operating principles, frequent user errors, patient adverse reactions, common reasons for mechanical failure, and emergency operations.

Nursing has traditionally made very little allowance for the insecurity of the new graduate. Creative approaches to easing the transition from student to professional should be formally endorsed by organized nursing. Work-study programs create comfort with practice (assuming, of course, that the work is nursing). Academically endorsed placement of students with affiliate agencies for summer work and part-time employment during the school year are another option. Postgraduate residencies or externships as part of the educational program should also be a consideration. Such arrangements require many decisions. Should they be mandatory or permissive? Who should control the educational program or service? Should participants be compensated?

The delivery of health care has shifted significantly from institutions to community-based settings. It is difficult to predict whether the market for nursing services will flow in the direction of these broader utilization patterns. An ANA/AMA paper on the future demand for health care predicts that there will be a 300 percent increase in the volume of home care delivered by the time the full effect of the Medicare prospective pricing system is felt (ANA, 1984). The "quicker and sicker" phenomenon has resulted in a dramatic increase in referrals to home care; however, there has not been a comparable increase in the utilization of registered nurses in the home. Home care aides and a vast variety of technicians and therapists dominate the home health scene (Joel, 1985).

According to ANA statistics, in 1970 approximately 5 percent of employed nurses worked in community settings (school nurses excluded). By 1980, the percentage had risen to 6.6, but in 1986 only 6.8 percent of nurses were employed in the community (C. Johnson, personal communication, 1985). These statistics reflect employment patterns two full years after the initiation of Medicare prospective pricing, which forced a dramatic shift to home care. Community practice in its many forms currently represents an underserved and undeveloped market for nurses. In many instances, community practice minimizes some of the variables that have significantly contributed to an impoverished work environment for nurses, such as autonomy constraints, physician domination, and direct access to clients. The Community Nursing Services and Ambulatory Care Act of 1987, presently before the 100th Congress, enables reimbursement to nurses under part B of Medicare without physician supervision or prescription (ANA, February 1987). The future looks bright for this legislation. If it is passed and fully implemented, it could establish community practice as the ideal employment setting for nurses.

In response to fairly obvious trends, clinical placements in community settings should be a major orientation of the curriculum. It should be noted that most faculty, except for those with a specialty in community or public health, have been socialized to hospital practice. Further, community nursing has been depicted as a practice area that first requires experience in hospital practice. These biases are conveyed both subtly and directly to students by faculty.

In reality, reimbursement models of the future are moving towards capitated systems that will limit both community and institutional resources. High acuity will continue to characterize the consumer in the health care delivery system. Fragmentation and complexity will pose a constant threat to continuity and comprehensive care. Rewards will be offered for self-care and the supplementary use of services provided by friends, family, and volunteers; it is logical that care is given most carefully by those who care. Service integration and coordination will cut costs and become desirable, if not essential. Provider professionals who can develop resources that do not add to the cost of the system will move into controlling positions. Client advocacy will be visible and valued by the consumer, who in fact has become the most significant player in the health care game. The role components described here—resource development, coordination, advocacy—are descriptive of the services that nurses have historically provided. If pieces have slipped from our grasp, they must be reclaimed.

Nursing is complicated by the presence of a work force with a variety of skill levels. Given the growing number of chronically ill and frail elderly, there are many lower-level activities in a plan of care that self-care and family cannot accomplish but that must be done. We are confronted with a future in which registered nurses will be responsible for care but in many institutions will delegate activities. Quick interpretation may create the picture of a return to outmoded models of supervision—layer on layer of people watching one another. Cost-consciousness is promoting new and better uses of the lesser skills of nursing aides, volunteers, and even patients themselves and their families. Industrial psychology has created a large body of knowledge in human resource development. The modus operandi has become to work with people to get them to internalize those values that are held by the leader in a system or philosophically established by the system. The system may be the client, the hospital, the home health agency, the primary nurse, or all of the above. Once subordinates understand and internalize these values, the amount of supervision that they require is reduced (Naisbitt & Aburdene, 1985). A natural first step towards helping others to internalize values is to clarify one's own values.

The theme that is emerging is one of decentralization of decisions to each registered nurse and personal accountability of registered nurses for the actions of ancillary workers. We need assertive people who have broad shoulders rather than strong backs. Since this delegation often requires decisions about the appropriate skill level for a given situation, clincial sophistication and comfort with research findings are critical. Practice based on outcomes and cost factors and a commitment to peer review should be established early in the educational program. Every ministration and design element in care should be tracked to its ultimate outcome and should be assessed in terms of cost and quality. Peer review should be a regular component of clinical conferencing. Students should continually evaluate one another as peers at similar levels of development. Computer literacy and a healthy respect for documentation go hand in hand with this expanded responsibility. Reimbursement and judgments on quality flow from the record. It is no secret that since the inception of Medicare prospective pricing, medical records has become the most powerful department in the hospital.

Emergent practice roles as described in this paper force us to admit that the setting for clinical experiences is less important than the role models provided and the role behaviors allowed. Faculty are not the role models for students, except in those rare instances in which faculty teach on their own panel of patients. Although faculty practice is the ultimate aim of many education–service collaborative efforts, many have lost sight of this mission over time. One of the most successful and emotionally uplifting aspects of the Rutgers Teaching Nursing Home Project has been the rich learning experiences students gain from being assigned directly to registered nurses employed at the home. Those nurses, who had a wide variety of entry-level preparations, were quick to encourage students to test their clinical and management skills. The nurses welcomed students' help in evaluating ancillary workers and making decisions on appropriate delegation. At first, when students were allowed a choice of clinical placements, they were reluctant to select experience based in a nursing home. In time, however, a waiting list had to be established for placement in the Teaching Nursing Home. Students reported the Teaching Nursing Home as the clinical experience most relevant to their world of work.

The rising acuity of hospital patients has renewed interest in the use of service agency staff as preceptors to students. It is almost impossible for a single instructor to supervise the activities of ten students who are taking care of extremely ill patients requiring highly complex care. This statement is not meant to challenge the 1/10 instructor/student ratio that is required by regulation in many states, merely to suggest that the use of staff as auxiliary teachers and preceptors should be maximized. There is the constant assumption that faculty are on site and in control. In addition, the art and science of clinical teaching lie in the case presentation and anlysis, which takes place in pre- and postclinical conference. I have observed that staff rise to the occasion and profit psychologically, attitudinally, and technically from being selected to work with students. Professionals have traditionally assumed responsibility for neophytes entering their field. In seeking to divorce ourselves from our roots, we have rejected many good aspects of apprenticeship education.

We artfully hide the fact that a great diversity of roles is inherent in a nursing career. Nurses need not commit their lives to direct patient care in order to contribute to the world of nursing. For example, positions in utilization review and case coordination are uniquely suited to nurses. Nurses are needed in government, organizational work, and other areas. Unfortunately, nurses are quick to criticize one another. Attraction to an atypical nursing role is often misconstrued as failure to survive in nursing. Nurses should be encouraged to pursue new roles, claim them for nurses and nursing, and use them as a platform to serve as advocates for their colleagues.

The contemporary roles available to nurses demand the substance of a true professional. The breadth of a liberal education and the depth of professional socialization are both essential to successful role execution. Existing practice opportunities should cause nursing leaders to reconsider traditional curriculum designs. The distaste for a layered educational experience should be temporarily put aside to allow reassessment. A preprofessional program that is rich in the natural and behavioral sciences and the humanities may provide an excellent base for the subsequent intense study of nursing. Socialization into the field may be the single most important goal of professional education. The educational patterns of law and medicine have been successful in developing professional identity, self-esteem, and collegial feeling. The nature and length of the preprofessional sequence have both educational and political implications, and they remain to be decided. The preprofessional requirement could be two years (an associate degree), or it could be patterned on existing master's level entry into practice programs. The ultimate result of health care restructuring may be a market for fewer but more sophisticated registered nurses.

SUMMARY AND CONCLUSIONS

Health care in the 1980s invites nurses to assume a more vigorous and visible leadership role. Traditional practice has become more complex, and new gaps in services exist that nurses are uniquely suited to fill. There are promising opportunities that could attract the best and the brightest into nursing.

Education for practice must highlight clinical placements that predict the future job market. Equally important is the presence of role models whom students would seek to emulate. The entry-level curriculum should convey the ethos of personal accountability for one's own practice and for ancillary personnel. Conscious acceptance of this responsibility will bring nurses one step closer to controlling the practice environment instead of being controlled by it.

Nursing is not unique in being threatened by a loss of control. Rapidly expanding technology and the limited shelflife of knowledge are a challenge to all the applied sciences. Nursing education can defend itself in part by ensuring beginning competency with medical devices. Further, a course of studies should consist of content that is selective, conceptual, and process-oriented. Educators must resist the temptation to "teach it all." Clinical material should rarely be used for its own sake; instead, it should be considered a vehicle for developing the cognitive processes that characterize the professional.

REFERENCES

American Nurses' Association. (1984, September). ANA's concerns regarding the impact of the prospective financing mechanisms on nursing service: ANA/AMA Joint Meeting. Kansas City, MO: Author.

American Nurses' Association. (1985). *Facts about nursing.* Kansas City, MO: Author.

American Nurses' Association. (1985, February). Introduction of community nursing organizations legislation. (Available from American Nurses' Association, Washington Office)

American Nurses' Association. (1985, July). *National public opinion survey on nursing.* Kansas City, MO: Author.

Green, K. C. (1987, March). Keynote presentation delivered at the 1987 semiannual meeting of the American Association of Colleges of Nursing, Washington, DC

Joel, L. (1985). *Nursing's role in the changing health scene.* Seattle: University of Washington School of Nursing.

Joel, L. (1987, June). Reshaping nursing practice. *American Journal of Nursing, 87*(6), 793–795.

Naisbitt, J. & Aburdene, P. (1985). *Reinventing the corporation.* New York: Warner.

"New York Hospital on the Spot". (1987, June 22) *New York Magazine,* pp. 40–47.

Pinchot, G. (1985). *Intrapreneuring.* New York: Harper & Row.

"The Debate: Shortage of Nurses." (1987, August 20). *USA Today.*

PROVIDING FACULTY DEVELOPMENT PROGRAMS ABOUT COMPUTER TECHNOLOGY ON A REGIONAL BASIS

Audrey F. Spector, MS, RN
Nursing Programs Director
Southern Regional Education Board
Atlanta, GA

Kathleen J. Mikan, PhD, RN
Professor and Director of Learning Resources
School of Nursing
University of Alabama at Birmingham

The rapidly growing use of computer technology in general education and in clinical areas makes it imperative that faculty in college-based nursing programs gain knowledge and skill in the use of such technology. In response to this growing need, the Southern Regional Education Board (SREB) submitted a proposal and was awarded a Nursing Special Projects grant by the Division of Nursing, Health Resources and Services Administration, Public Health Service, U. S. Department of Health and Human Services. The aim of the proposal was to promote systematic implementation of computer-supported nursing education in undergraduate nursing programs in the South. Computer-supported nursing education is defined in this project as the use of computers within an educational setting to facilitate the achievement of the organization's goals, purposes, and functions. This term is broad in scope and includes diverse applications of computers (both microcomputers and mainframe computers) in teaching, research, communication, data processing, and administration. The project addressed the diverse applications of computers in nursing education, not just computer-assisted instruction. The continuing education project, which began on March 1, 1985, focuses on faculty teaching in undergraduate nursing programs, specifically in institutions offering associate degree programs, baccalaureate programs, or both.

The project is administered by SREB, the first interstate compact for higher education in the United States. Its central concern is the optimum use of higher education resources in the Southern region. The 15 member states are Alabama, Arkansas, Florida, Georgia, Kentucky, Louisiana, Maryland, Mississippi, North Carolina, Oklahoma, South Carolina, Tennessee, Texas, Virginia, and West Virginia. The project is implemented in cooperation with the Southern Council on Collegiate Education for Nursing, a regional nursing group consisting of 222 institutions in the SREB states.

The members of the project staff are Audrey F. Spector (program director), Eula Aiken (project director), and Delena T. Martin (project secretary). Kathleen J. Mikan (University of Alabama at Birmingham School of Nursing) is the project consultant and assisted in the development of the proposal.

The major goal of the project is to provide continuing education about computer technology for nursing faculty in 430 collegiate nursing programs in the 15 Southern states. Specifically, the project was designed to strengthen the ability of over 5,000 nurse faculty in undergraduate collegiate programs to use computer technology as an instructional tool.

The grant provided multiple and diverse educational opportunities, including decentralized basic workshops, seminars, regional conferences, and networking opportunities. An advisory committee, appointed in March 1985, provides input on plans for the conferences and seminars. The members of the committee are Cora Balmat (Alcorn State University, Natchez, Mississippi), Carol Buisson (Louisiana State University Medical Center), Barbara Brown (Vanderbilt University, Nashville, Tennessee), Richard E. Pogue (Pogue Associates, Ltd., Augusta, Georgia), and Elizabeth Wajdowicz (St. Petersburg Junior College, St. Petersburg, Florida).

DESCRIPTION OF ACTIVITIES

Several types of project activities are being implemented in the project. These are described briefly below.

Basic Workshops

The workshops were designed as basic educational experiences for nurse faculty who have little or no previous training in or experience with computer technology as an instructional tool. The workshops are offered at six different host sites, each of which is within reasonable driving distance of large numbers of nursing faculty. Host sites were selected on the basis of geographic location, access to computer resources, and availability of people with experience in using the technology. The following are the host institutions (the coordinator is in parentheses):

- Virginia Commonwealth University, MCV School of Nursing (Linda L. Lange);

- University of South Carolina (Columbia), College of Nursing (Mary Ann Schroeder);
- University of Florida, College of Nursing (Margaret Wilson);
- University of Alabama at Birmingham, School of Nursing (Kathleen C. Brown);
- University of Tennessee, Memphis, College of Nursing (Donna Hathaway); and
- University of Texas Medical Branch (Galveston), School of Nursing (Douglas Haskin).

The six coordinators play a major role in conducting the basic workshops. All are knowledgeable about and experienced with computers. The nurse administrative head at each institution provides release time to allow the coordinators to plan and conduct the workshops.

A single master plan (including objectives and program outline) for the five two-day workshops to be conducted at the host institutions and for common evaluation tools is used at all sites. This plan is based on a conceptual model for systematic implementation of computer-supported nursing education developed by Dr. Mikan. Each of the five workshops has its own theme:

1. Moving into the age of computer-supported nursing education;
2. Computers as instructional tools;
3. Software selection, production, and evaluation;
4. Special computer applications in nursing education; and
5. Managing computer-supported education.

The workshops are planned as a series, with each building on the preceding ones. Individuals are encouraged to attend the entire series of five workshops; however, for practical reasons, attendance at previous workshops is not a requirement. Workshop dates are determined by each host institution; and SREB promotes the workshops with brochures throughout the region. All of the scheduled five workshops have now been implemented; the last was offered during the fall of 1987.

The site coordinators, in conjunction with local resource persons from the community or institution hosting the workshop, conduct the basic workshops. Additional local resource persons are invited to participate as needed to achieve the specific objectives of each workshop; these may include programmers, curriculum specialists, and nurses from local health care agencies using computers. Opportunities are provided for the participants to have structured and unstructured hands-on experiences. During the workshops, many faculty review software programs already purchased by the host institutions. Under the aegis of the Georgia Nurses' Association, SREB awards nine contact hours to the participants who complete each two-day workshop.

The basic workshops are popular among the faculty. All together, more than 500 people have participated. The coordinators meet periodically to plan the implementation of the basic workshops so that there is consistency between the content and learning activities provided at each site.

Seminars

A total of four one-day seminars are planned for individuals who already know the basics of computer technology and have more experience in computer instruction. The purpose of the seminars is to facilitate discussion of critical issues related to instructional computer programs. A three-day seminar was held at Alcorn State University (Natchez, Mississippi) in May 1986. The title of the seminar was "Forecasting Excellence in Computer Programs for Nursing Education." Issues surrounding "quality instructional software" were the foci of the presentations and group discussions. The following were among the questions addressed:

1. What is the current status of software evaluation?
2. What is quality software?
3. How should nurse educators evaluate software? and
4. What can we do to influence change in the quality?

Among the 62 attendees at the seminar were deans or directors of nursing programs, persons responsible for computer-assisted instruction, directors of learning resource centers, and representatives from state boards of nursing. The two major outcomes of this seminar were (1) a draft evaluation tool for instructional software specific to nursing and (2) a definition of quality instructional software. Quality software is defined as a computer program that provides a purposeful, valued, well-designed, interactive, content-accurate, motivational learning experience that capitalizes on the potentials of the computer, responds to a variety of user input, and facilitates the achievement of desirable predetermined outcomes by a target population efficiently, effectively, and creatively.

The draft evaluation tool, which was circulated to the college-based nursing programs in the South for review and use on a trial basis, was revised at another seminar in April 1987. The focus of the April seminar, held at SREB headquarters in Atlanta, Georgia, was software evaluation. Its primary purpose, under the leadership of Linda Speranza (Valencia Community College), was to review and revise the draft evaluation tool. Other nurse educators involved in the revision were Kathleen C. Brown (Alabama), Frances Henderson (Mississippi), Kathleen J. Mikan (Alabama), Marilyn Ann Murphy (Texas), Rose Marie Norris (Georgia), Maribeth K. Traer (Virginia), and Carol Wiggs (Texas). The revised form is designed to help faculty overcome major obstacles to the evaluation, selection, and use of instructional software.

Nearly 100 nurse educators expressed interest in a seminar on instructional software development that was held at Louisiana State Medical Center School of Nursing (New Orleans) in May 1987. The format of the seminar limited the number of participants to 34. Under the leadership of Richard Pogue, this seminar provided an opportunity for nurse educators to discuss and practice basic steps in the development of instructional software using an authoring system.

Regional Conferences

Regional conferences are designed to allow greater intraregional faculty involvement and interchange among the schools. They also provide opportunities to invite speakers outside the SREB region; for example, Donna Larson (Michigan) and Sheila Ryan (New York) shared their knowledge and experiences at the first regional conference, held in Atlanta, Georgia, in October 1986. In addition to the featured speakers and group activities, participants at the regional conferences can browse through the "marketplace," where books and other materials are displayed. Representatives from several publishing companies have been available to discuss software selections.

Networking

A goal of the project is to increase networking within the region. The following activities help promote achievement of this goal:

- Planned times and activities for networking are built into the workshop, seminar, and conference agenda; for example, workshop participants shared "success stories" at several of the workshops.

- A regional newsletter is published for the purposes of sharing and disseminating information about the project. It includes highlights of information presented at basic workshops, seminars, and conferences.

- A Resource Directory identifies individuals in the region with experience in using computers who want to network with other nurse educators. In addition to a roster of educators, the directory (revised in April 1987) includes the names of speakers at basic workshops, along with selected references and publications.

Although many of the networking opportunities are preplanned, some networking occurs spontaneously in response to the environment. An evening dinner on a Mississippi river boat provided a ideal place for attendees to network informally and added considerably to the enjoyment of the seminar at Alcorn State University.

EVALUATION

Evaluation is a crucial part of this project. Each workshop is evaluated by the participants, by the site coordinators, and by the project staff. The participant is asked to complete a participant's Profile Form at the first workshop attended. This instrument provides information about the person's level of expertise in and use of computers, as well as information about the computer involvement at the participant's institution. At the end of each basic workshop, participants complete a workshop evaluation form and a Plan to Enhance form that identifies specific computer implementation activities to be accomplished during the interval between workshops. (Some participants from the same institution work as a team on this Plan.) A dominant theme in the plans is the need for faculty development activities to help faculty become proficient in the use of computers. A six-month progress report form is mailed to all participants to determine how each has used the workshop information. Responses on the returns indicate that the educators are using the information and materials distributed at workshops.

Several articles have been published as a result of the workshops and seminars, and others are being prepared. Project-related articles have appeared in *Computers in Nursing* and *The Journal of Continuing Education in Nursing*.

Summaries of the data collected from workshop participants are a rich source of "implementation data." These summaries provide insight into faculty needs, goals, activities, and institutional resources. The progress reports provide information about the types of problems encountered, outcomes achieved, unintended outcomes, and facilitating factors. The project has generated a wealth of data about the process of using computer technology in nursing education.

A prepost assessment instrument was developed and administered to 424 college-based nursing programs in the region to collect baseline data about the use of computer technology in undergraduate nursing programs. The response rate to the prequestionnaire was 75 percent. The data have been tabulated and analyzed in terms of (1) direct and indirect uses of microcomputers within schools of nursing and (2) the extent of implementation of computers within undergraduate curriculum.

OUTCOMES

The impact of this continuing education project has been documented in progress reports and the Plans submitted by faculty who participated in various activities. Faculty have experienced successes as well as problems when implementing computer-supported education within their institutions.

At the completion of the project, the master plan for the basic decentralized workshops will be made available for other institutions to use or modify to meet their needs. The evaluation instruments and the entire process for conducting the project will be published and made available for others to use.

SUMMARY

This three-year project provides basic decentralized continuing education workshops for faculty in college-based nursing programs in the South. It also offers seminars and conferences and disseminates information about computer-related activities. This is the only regional faculty development effort being implemented at this time. The process, methods, and instruments used in this project will be available to other groups and should assist them in developing educational programs to enhance faculty use of computer technology in nursing education.

EVALUATING ADMINISTRATORS
IN SCHOOLS OF NURSING

Gaye W. Poteet, EdD, RN
Assistant Dean of Graduate Program
and Professor, School of Nursing
East Carolina University
Greenville, NC

The 1980s are going to be remembered as a time when social and economic policy profoundly influenced both higher education and nursing education. Rapid social change and the economic reality of an overwhelming national deficit brought about changes in the financing of health care that forever changed the way we manage that industry. All of the changes in our society have forced nursing educators, as a professional group, to reexamine what administrative skills are needed and wanted.

The changes in health care and society have in fact brought about a need for nursing leaders who can react appropriately to change and who can lead their schools of nursing through troubled times marked by declining student enrollments. One study conducted by Arthur Anderson and Company found that the skills needed by future chief executive officers of institutions will undergo a major change, with financial management and strategic planning skills becoming the most important skills for executives (American Hospital Association, 1984). For some schools, the quality of the leadership will determine whether or not the school of nursing continues to exist.

Nursing education has been a growth industry for several decades. Few faculty members or administrators in the public sector have prior experience with large decreases in student enrollment and the subsequent need to downsize the operation. *Financial exigency* and *retrenchment* are familiar terms to many in higher education; however, faculty in the health professions, including nursing, have until now been largely exempt from the financial realities of declining student enrollment.

The 1960s and 1970s were marked by increased enrollments in existing nursing schools and the establishment of new nursing schools at what seemed like every crossroads in America. The reality of those decades was that the institution and the nursing program would succeed and perhaps even prosper, regardless of the quality of leadership in the nursing unit. Today, however, survival of the university and of selected schools or programs in nursing is no longer assured. In fact, it is estimated that by the year 1995, 10 to 30 percent of the 3,100 universities and colleges will have closed their doors or merged with other institutions (Keller, 1983, p. 3).

Colleges, universities, and, more recently, hospitals across the country are closing their doors in ever-increasing numbers. In many instances, these institutions are closing their doors because of the quality of the leadership that was in place. The type of leadership necessary for survival in a growth industry fueled by capitation monies presents a very different set of requirements than does that necessary for successfully competing in a climate characterized by intense competition at all levels.

Survival, even in prestigious schools of nursing, now requires educational administrators who are able to position their schools and programs favorably in the competitive marketing arena. Strategic and successful marketing of all school programs is vital in today's climate. It was much easier to be a successful educational administrator when the students and the monies were pouring in.

REASONS FOR ADMINISTRATIVE EVALUATION

During these times of declining student enrollment in schools of nursing and accompanying faculty layoffs, faculty are not as willing to exempt their leaders from careful examination of performance and productivity. Some administrators and faculty express the view that a basic conceptual problem exists with administrators being evaluated from below. This argument is a difficult one to support, when students have long evaluated their professors from below. In 1973, the higher education community's attention was called to the obvious parallel between student evaluation of faculty and faculty evaluation of administrators:

> If teachers can be aided by securing systematically the ratings of their students it follows logically that administrators also may be helped in improving their work by obtaining ratings from the persons with whom they deal most directly—the academic faculty. Some administrators will deny the usefulness of such ratings, as many teachers oppose, for various reasons, the idea of being evaluated by their students. Since teacher-ratings scales have become widely accepted, however, there seems little reason to doubt the eventual acceptance in higher education of rating scales for academic administrators. (Hillway, 1973)

Further support for evaluation of educational administrators seems likely in the context of the current environment in which nursing education must operate.

The implementation of any form of administrative evaluation is a source of concern to all those who must participate. If the plan can be conceptualized and implemented during a time in which the school is relatively free of conflict, all parties are better served. Unfortunately, cries for the implementation of administrator evaluation can signal serious discontent and unrest within a school. When this situation exists, it is difficult for all parties to cooperate in an unbiased program of administrative evaluation. Administrative evaluation, like other aspects of the school evaluation program, is most successful when the goal is a careful assessment of efficiency and effectiveness with no hidden agendas.

There are many pros and cons that can be expressed in support of or in opposition to administrator evaluation. In today's competitive environment, however, it is very difficult to come up with a sound rationale for failure to evaluate the schools' leadership, for in many ways the performance of a nursing school's leadership is the most important factor in determining the future of the school.

Furthermore, nursing educators have long exhibited an almost fanatical devotion to the evaluation of their programs, including their students. Evaluations given by other groups of educators do not begin to approximate the breadth and scope of evaluations given by nursing school educators. In fact, when other university professors are confronted with evaluation programs in schools of nursing, they are often astonished at the scope and extent of the programs. With this evaluation obsession (or heritage, depending on one's point of view), it is difficult to imagine allowing nursing school administrators to escape the process.

In summary, nursing educators generally want their administrators to be evaluated, and the majority of administrators are willing to be evaluated; however, both groups express their misgivings about actual participation in the administrative evaluation process and the long-term viability of the process in their school of nursing. The majority of faculty indicate that they support some type of administrative evaluation. Where the differences and the difficulties arise is in determining what administrator evaluation is, what elements are important to include, and what the measures of administrative productivity are (in other words, what makes an administrator successful or unsuccessful in today's world).

REVIEW OF LITERATURE

A selective review of the literature on administrative evaluation reveals a variety of publications, which can be classified into the following categories:

1. The administrative evaluation process in higher education,

2. Reports on evaluation instruments and role scales, and

3. The administrative evaluation process in schools of nursing.

During the 1970s, articles about administrative evaluation in higher education began appearing in the literature. In many of the references, the need for administrative evaluation was linked to the declining numbers of college students and the resulting financial exigency (Farmer, 1979; Fisher, 1978; Anderson, 1976; Nordvall, 1977). Other authors urged the higher education community and faculty members in particular to recognize the potential contributions the evaluation process can make to the improvement of educational services (Dresssel, 1976; Miller, 1979). Other writers proposed programs to help administrators improve the effectiveness of their work (Hillway, 1973; Zion, 1977).

Reports on evaluation instruments and rating scales appeared in numerous publications (Hillway, 1973; Sapone, 1980; Gasmussen, 1978; Brown, 1978; Turner, 1974). One classic reference (Genova, Madoff, Chin, & Thomas, 1976) presents in book form a comprehensive approach to the evaluation of faculty and administrators.

Administrative evaluation in schools of nursing appears to be in an even earlier developmental stage than administrative evaluation in higher education in general (Rozendal, 1977). In her dissertation research, Rozendal reported an absence of any previous studies on the evaluation of educational administrators in nursing. She surveyed the 170 administrators of all the accredited baccalaureate nursing education programs in the United States and found that there was both an absence of formal administrative evaluation and a lack of interest in being evaluated on the part of school of nursing administrators. She also found that the most common method of evaluation is an evaluation by superiors.

A study (Fenneran, 1983) that surveyed a random sample of the membership of the American Association of Colleges of Nursing indicated a trend toward some form of administrative evaluation of deans and directors. The sample subjects (deans) reported that the dean's evaluations were initiated by anyone or by a combination of the following: the dean herself, her immediate superiors, the president, or the faculty.

Formal evaluation procedures existed in 38 (60 percent) of the institutions surveyed. There was general agreement that the purpose of administrative evaluation was to assess the dean's overall performance. The most frequently cited criteria for evaluation were productivity, effectiveness, performance in the role, leadership, and management skills (Fenneran, 1983).

The primary response of the most current study concerned with administrative evaluation (Hodges & Christ, 1987) was to describe current methods of administrative evaluation in schools of nursing. Four hundred seventy-eight National League for Nursing-accredited schools were surveyed. The study findings indicated that unit administrators in private institutions were younger and less experienced and had been in their positions longer than their counterparts in public institutions. Administrative evaluation was found to be based on job descriptions, governed by formal policies, and conducted on an annual basis.

PURPOSES OF ADMINISTRATIVE EVALUATION

The purposes of administrative evaluation are outlined in several different ways in the literature. Statements of purpose can be adapted for use in the school evaluation plans, with citations providing credit to the originator and author. One classic reference on administrative evaluation (Farmer, 1979), which is applicable to nursing education as it was to higher education, states that administrative evaluation has the following three purposes:

1. To identify and anticipate changes in the perceptions and values in the institution or its constituencies;
2. To measure the impact of administrative behavior on the school's efficiency and effectiveness; and
3. To relate administrative action to organizational policy in order to ensure compatibility between individual, institutional, and school goals.

In this view, a program of administrative evaluation is needed to provide the school of nursing with the data necessary to achieve these purposes.

A more specific listing of the purposes of administrative evaluation was offered by another group of writers (Thomas et al, 1977):

1. Establishing and attaining institutional goals;
2. Helping individual administrators to improve their performance;
3. Making decisions on retention, salary, or promotion;
4. Increasing the effectiveness and efficiency of the administration as a team;
5. Keeping an inventory of personnel resources for reassignment or retraining;
6. Informing the governing body and administration of the degree of congruence between institutional policy and institutional action;
7. Sharing governance;
8. Informing internal and external audiences about administrative effectiveness and worth; and
9. Conducting research on factors related to administrative effectiveness.

Although not all of these purposes are likely to be appropriate for use in every school of nursing, the list can serve as a checklist for guiding faculty as they seek to articulate the desired outcomes of the administrative evaluation program.

It seems feasible to incorporate administrative evaluation into an existing systematic plan of program evaluation in one of two ways. Either it can be added to an existing section or administration, or a separate section or category can be added. As should be done with any addition or change in the overall evaluation plan, the calendar must be revised to reflect the changes and the proposed timetable. The leader is referred to an earlier conference on program evaluation for a more in-depth discussion of program evaluation (Poteet & Pollok, 1986).

WHO PARTICIPATES IN ADMINISTRATOR EVALUATION?

The appropriate participants in administrative evaluation are the administrator being reviewed, faculty, senior administrators, staff and support personnel, and, in some instances, students. Committee evaluations or task force members are advised to answer the question of who should evaluate school administrators. When this question is addressed early in the deliberations, the remaining work can proceed more logically. The goal of the group is the incorporation of all school elements, including administration/leadership, into the overall evaluation plan, with the group's ultimate goal being the advancement of the school of nursing.

The participation of faculty in administrative evaluation is an issue on which administrators differ. Nonetheless, faculty assessment of the effectiveness or ineffectiveness of administrative performance is probably the most important aspect of administrative evaluation. When faculty fail to support the administrator, that lack of support is indicative of a troubled school environment. An evaluation system that includes both upward and downward evaluation assures both groups of feedback on their performance.

Another important reference on administrative evaluation (Anderson, 1976) graphically describes the importance of the faculty viewpoint:

> Faculty members carry the value system of the college or university; i.e., they are the institution in terms of performance, values, interactions, meaning, significance, and, in the end, they satisfy that crass word, productivity. While faculty can on occasion be insensitive, even cruel, they must tell it as they perceive it regarding academic administrators. If an administrator is brilliant, let the faculty say so; if shabby, let them report it in the same fashion. They should be guided by their professionalism and by their professional or disciplinary perspectives and commitments. They should be forthright, open, and, if necessary, courageous in making their evaluations. (Anderson, 1976)

DIMENSIONS OF ADMINISTRATIVE EVALUATION

The articles and books on administrative evaluation agree on why evaluation should be done, but not on what should be evaluated. Questions are likely to be raised concerning criteria and the qualities or areas of administrative performance that can be evaluated by faculty. A program of administrative evaluation requires that a plan or model be developed that identifies the competencies and expectations inherent in each administrative position. The areas of administrative behavior that constitute this model (see Table 1) are leadership, management, quality of work, membership satisfaction, professional commitment, institutional commitment, and personal integrity. Although the model is not a replication of any earlier work, its development was influenced by the review of previous administrative evaluation plans and the work of numerous authors on the subject. The most significant influence on the model was Helsabeck's (1973) article describing a framework for evaluating the effectiveness of administrative performance, In this framework, the evaluation of the administrator is based on successful performance in the areas of goal formation, goal attainment, resource acquisition, and membership satisfaction. The framework of the model was also influenced by the conceptualization of leadership and management developed and described by Bennis and Nanus (1986).

Since administrators in schools of nursing share job expectations with administrators and managers in other fields, it seemed appropriate to incorporate concepts from these works that have been found to be useful; however, the dimensions for administrator evaluation in schools of nursing shown in Table 1 were specifically developed and conceptualized for use in schools of nursing. Faculty are encouraged to use the plan as desired in their individual schools. The administrator evaluation form is shown in full in Figure 1 to facilitate its use in schools of nursing. Individual groups may also wish to alter the instrument scale used in this plan; some schools prefer a seven-point scale rather than a five-point one.

The size of the organization, the actual number of administrators, and the complexity of their jobs most often determine whether it is preferable to design a system that evaluates all administrators on the same dimensions or to develop unique dimensions and evaluation tools for individual administrators. In most schools of nusing, the most reasonable approach seems to be a single set of job dimensions that is based on a careful review of job expectations and existing job descriptions.

The overall goal of administrtive evaluation remains the same, regardless of program size, type, and complexity. It has been described as follows:

> The primary goal of administrator evaluation as previously stated is to improve organization effectiveness and efficiency which translates into

monitoring and improving the quality of teaching, all areas of scholarship, including the conduct of research and practice and community service. Unlike faculty, administrators generally have little direct contact
with students and may not be expected to engage in ongoing research.
Therefore, a program of administrator evaluation must be designed to
measure the administrator's contributions to the school of nursing and
the university as a whole. (Poteet, in press)

Emphasis and job requirements vary from one school of nursing to another.
The program described above was designed to be sufficiently broad in scope
to be usable in multiple situations, including all types of nursing programs.
In each situation, however, individuals are advised to consider carefully the
elements of each dimension of administrative evaluation. Elements that are
not applicable can be discarded, and those job components that are missing
from this plan can be added.

Table 1. Dimensions of Administrator Evaluation*

Leadership
Strategic planning, vision
Social and political realities
Group interest and pressures
Ability to initiate new ideas and changes
Professional appearance

Management
Financial skills—careful and sound fiscal management, ability to attract
    money for institution
Operational planning
Resource acquisition, human and material
    Ability to allocate resources
    Ability to select strong subordinates
    Ability to delegate
    Evaluation program and successes in planning
Decision-making skills, including ability to incorporate ideas of others
Assign work fairly and appropriately

Quality of work
Knowledge of nursing and administration
Organized
Adaptable
Meets deadlines
Judgment

Membership satisfaction (interpersonal relationships)
Impartial in relationships with faculty, staff, and students
Considerate of faculty, staff, and students
Readily approachable
Receptive to new ideas

Professional commitment
Understands role of politics and government
Awareness of issues and trends in nursing and higher education
Contributes to knowledge development in field
Commitment to excellence in teaching, scholarship, practice, and community
    service
Continued professional development

Institutional commitment
Well-developed goals and objectives
Academic evaluation program
Ability to work with other university officials
Ability to inititate curricular changes
Skills in relating to university, community, alumni, and board

Personal integrity
Assumes responsibility for actions
Adheres to decisions of group
Fair and impartial
Trustworthiness
Respects professional and legal rights of faculty, staff, and students

*From Poteet, *Nursing Outlook* (article in press).

Figure 1. Administrator Evaluation Questionnaire

Name of Individual evaluated: _____

   Position: _____

Your status: Faculty ☐   Administrator ☐   Staff ☐   Student ☐

Directions: Listed below are statements describing administrator behavior. Rate your administrator on each item by marking the appropriate response.

Dimension I: Leadership

	Superior	Above Average	Average	Below Average	Poor
1. Receptive to new ideas					
2. Ability to bring about group action					
3. Appropriate dress and grooming					
4. Ability to inspire confidence					
5. Gives generous credit to others for their ideas and contributions					
6. Encourages initiative and innovation					
7. Helps others to develop their full potential					
8. Clearly states goals for the future					

Dimension II: Management

	Superior	Above Average	Average	Below Average	Poor
1. Prepares appropriate budget					
2. Able to negotiate successfully for resources					
3. Adapts school plans to meet changing needs and demands					
4. Ability to allocate resources equitably and efficiently					
5. Recuits qualified middle and first-line school administrators					
6. Delegates effectively					
7. Maintains ongoing systematic evaluation program					
8. Incorporates evaluation findings into the decision-making process					
9. Provides leadership in curriclum process					
10. Approaches decision-making process in a systematic manner					
11. Gathers pertinent data before acting on a problem					
12. Confers with persons involved before acting on a problem					
13. Assigns work fairly and appropriately					
14. Maintains appropriate physical plant, equipment, and supplies					

(Continued next page)

Dimension III: Quality of Work

	Superior	Above Average	Average	Below Average	Poor
1. Knowledgeable about nursing and nursing education					
2. Plans, paces, and organizes the ongoing work of the organization					
3. Conducts meetings in an effective manner					
4. Meets deadlines					
5. Strives for excellence in all programs					
6. Maintains standards of appropriate professional organizations and regulatory bodies					
7. Communicates effectively					
8. Is accessible to faculty and students					

Dimension IV: Membership Satisfaction: Interpersonal Relationships

	Superior	Above Average	Average	Below Average	Poor
1. Is fair and impartial in relationships with faculty, staff, and students					
2. Gives public recognition and credit to others for their ideas and contributions					
3. Is receptive to new ideas and innovative approaches					
4. Is available and approachable					
5. Encourages discussion and debate					
6. Avoids retaliation and personal vendettas against selected faculty, students, and staff who may disagree or express unpopular opinions					
7. Demonstrates respect for individual employees					
8. Understands the total faculty role					
9. Develops faculty, staff, and students to full potential					
10. Provides for the mentoring of young or new faculty					

(Continued next page)

Dimension V: Professional Commitment

	Superior	Above Average	Average	Below Average	Poor
1. Understands the role of policies and government in nursing education					
2. Alert to issues and trends in higher education					
3. Recognizes the role of scholar within the faculty role					
4. Recognizes the role of scholar within the administrative role					
5. Contributes to knowledge development in nursing science					
6. Demonstrates commitment to teaching, research, practice, and community service					
7. Participates in appropriate professional development activities					
8. Maintains a leadership role in professional associations and organizations					

Dimension VI: Institutional Commitment

	Superior	Above Average	Average	Below Average	Poor
1. Has well-developed goals and objectives that support institutional aims and programs of the institution					
2. Participates in overall academic evaluation processes					
3. Ability to work harmoniously and effectively with university administrators					
4. Possesses ability to institute change					
5. Communicates effectively with university, community, alumni, and board representatives					
6. Promotes the image of the school of nursing and the parent institution					

(Continued next page)

Dimension VII: Personal Integrity

	Superior	Above Average	Average	Below Average	Poor
1. Assumes responsibility for decisions and action taken					
2. Respects and adheres to group decisions					
3. Maintains confidentiality					
4. Safeguards academic freedom					
5. Respects the professional and legal rights of faculty, staff, and students					

Questionnaire © 1987 by Gaye W. Poteet.

REFERENCES

American Hospital Association. (1984). *Health care in the 1990's: Trends and strategies.* Chicago, IL: Arthur Anderson & Company.

Anderson, G. (1976). *The evaluation of academic administrators: Principles, processes, and outcomes.* University Park: Center for The Study of Higher Education, The Pennsylvania State University.

Bennis, W., & Nanus, B. (1985). *Leaders: The strategies for taking charge.* New York: Harper & Row.

Brown, E. (1978). Faculty evaluation of administrators: The experience of Brooklyn College. *AAUP Bulletin, 64,* 298–304.

Dressel, P. (1976). *Handbook of academic evaluation.* San Francisco: Jossey-Bass.

Ezell, A., & Packard, J. (1985). An argument for the preparation of academic administrators in nursing. *Journal of Professional Nursing, 1*(3), 157–163.

Farmer, C. (Ed.). (1979). *Administrator evaluation: Concepts, methods, cases in higher education.* Richmond, VA: Higher Education Leadership and Management Society.

Featherstone, R., & Romano, L. (1977). Evaluation of adminstrative performance. *The Clearing House, 50*(9), 412–415.

Fenneran, M. (1983). Trends in the evaluation of nursing deans. *Nursing Outlook, 31*(3), 172–175.

Fisher, C. (Ed.). (1978). *Developing and evaluating administrative leadership.* San Francisco: Jossey-Bass.

Fisher, C. (1978). The evaluation and development of college and university administrators. In J. Shtogren (Ed.), *Administrative development in higher education.* Richmond, VA: Higher Education Leadership and Management Society.

Gasmussen, G. (1978). Evaluating the academic dean. *New Directions for Higher Education, 22,* 23–40.

Genova, W. J., Madoff, M. K., Chin, R., & Thomas, G. B. (1976). *Mutual benefit evaluation of faculty and administrators in higher education.* Cambridge, MA: Ballinger.

Helsabeck, R. E. (1973). *The compound system: A conceptual framework for effective decision making in colleges.* Berkeley, CA: Center for Research and Development in Higher Education, University of California.

Hillway, L. (1973). Evaluating college and university administrators. *Intellect, 101,* 426–427.

Hodges, L. C., & Christ, M. A. (1987). Variables influencing administrative evaluation of nursing deans and directors in public and private institutions. *Journal of Professional Nursing, 3*(2), 102–109.

Keller, G. (1983). *Academic strategy: The management revolution in American higher education.* Baltimore, MD: John Hopkins University Press.

Lucas, M. (1986). The relationship of nursing deans' leadership behaviors with institutional characteristics. *Journal of Nursing Education, 25*(2), 50–54.

Martin, E. (1983). New perspectives in educational selection of nursing deans. *Nursing Outlook, 31*(3), 168–172.

Miller, R. (1979). *The assessment of college performance.* San Francisco: Jossey-Bass.

Nordvall, R. (1979). *Evaluation and development of administrators.* Washington, DC: American Association of Higher Education.

Nordvall, R. C. (1977). Evaluation of college administrators: Where are we now? *NASPA Journal, 16*(2), 53–59.

Partridge, R. (1983). The decanal role: A dilemma of academic leadership. *Journal of Nursing Education, 22*(2), 59–61.

Pollok, C. S. (1983). Adapting management by objectives to nursing. *Nursing Clinics of North America, 18*(3), 481–490.

Poteet, G. W. (in press). Implementing administrative review in a school of nursing. *Nursing Outlook.*

Poteet, G. W., & Pollok, C. S. (1986). A model for program evaluation. *Nurse Educator, 11*(2), 41–47.

Reid, J. (1982). Politics and quality in administrative evaluation. *Research in Higher Education, 16*(1), 27–39.

Rozendal, N. (1977). *The evaluation of administrators of baccalaureate nursing programs: A study of current practices.* Unpublished doctoral dissertation, Boston University.

Sapone, C. (1980). An appraisal and evaluation system for teachers and administrators. *Educational Technology, 20*(5), 44–49.

Seldin, R. (1984). *Evaluating higher education.* Baltimore, MD: The University of Maryland, University College, Conferences and Institutes Program.

Stanton, M., & Styles, M. (1985). A phenomenological approach to understanding the process of deaning. *Journal of Professional Nursing, 1*(5), 269–274.

Thomas, G. B., Genova, W., Madoff, M., & Chin, R. (1977). Mutual benefit evaluation of administrators. *Journal of the College and University Personnel Association, 28*(3), 13–24.

Turner, L. (1984). Administrator evaluation. *Journal of the National School Development Council, 3*(3), 24–25.

Zion, C. (1977). Role definition: A focus for administrative growth and evaluation *Journal of the College and University Personnel Association, 28*(3), 5–12.

RESEARCH

MOVING NURSING RESEARCH
TO THE NATIONAL INSTITUTES OF HEALTH

Ada Sue Hinshaw, PhD, RN
Director, National Center for Nursing Research
National Institutes of Health
Bethesda, MD

Doris H. Merritt, MD
Director, Office of Extramural Research and Training
National Institutes of Health
Bethesda, MD

The basis for moving nursing research to the National Institutes of Health was the concept of incorporating nursing science into the broader base of other health care research. Bringing nursing research endeavors and programs into the visible health science structure—i.e., NIH—was believed to have several benefits. First, nursing research, with its orientation toward health promotion and disease prevention, as well as its emphasis on basic and clinical care processes, provided a natural complement to the biomedical research orientation that traditionally typifies NIH's research endeavors. Second, nursing science needed to be developed within the context of other basic and clinical health care disciplines. This would allow nursing research, which often draws on multiple bodies of knowledge from other fields, to be in contact with experts representing various sciences. In addition, as scientific knowledge was developed from the nursing perspective, it could be more visibly incorporated into health care knowledge in general and thus be more accessible to other disciplines as well as to our own. Third, moving nursing research into our nation's well-recognized structure for biomedical and behavioral research was expected to provide stability in resource allocation for nursing research, as it has for the research programs of other health care disciplines.

The following discussion of the move of the Center for Nursing Research to NIH will be divided into four parts:

1. The history of the establishment of the National Center for Nursing Research;

2. The mission of the NCNR in relationship to the mission of NIH;
3. The current structure and programs of NCNR; and
4. Future initiatives of the NCNR.

HISTORY OF THE ESTABLISHMENT OF NCNR

On April 18, 1986, the Secretary of Health and Human Services, Dr. Otis Bowen, announced the establishment of the National Center for Nursing Research within the National Institutes of Health. The NCNR had been authorized under the Health Research Extension Act of 1985 (Public Law 99-158). Dr. Doris H. Merritt was appointed acting director.

This final establishment of the NCNR was the result of a number of years of legislative activity, systematic study, and negotiations by nursing's professional organizations. The legislative initiative to create a national structure for nursing research within the NIH was partially motivated by the Institute of Medicine's 1983 study released on nursing and nursing education. In essence, the IOM study recommended that "the Federal Government should establish an organizational entity to place nursing research in the mainstream of scientific investigation. An adequately funded focal point is needed at the national level to foster research" (p. 19). This report formalized an issue raised by the Commission on Nursing Research of the American Nurses' Association in the 1970s, that is, the need to structure nursing research at the federal level with other health care sciences in order to stimulate investigator activity. Scientific growth would be enhanced by access to the rich multidisciplinary knowledge generated and shared within the health science structure of NIH and the security of a stable funding base.

The legislative endeavors began with the introduction by Representative Edward R. Madigan (R-Illinois) of a bill to amend the NIH reauthorization in 1983 to create a National Institute of Nursing within NIH. This bill was passed by the House of Representatives on November 17, 1983, but was pocket vetoed in October 1984. In vetoing the bill, President Reagan suggested that extending NIH at that time was not wise, because a study of the NIH structure had been undertaken by the IOM and was to be released shortly.

The 1984 IOM study of the NIH essentially recommended that any new institute in the NIH must meet several requirements:

- It must be compatible with the research and research training mission of the NIH;
- It must address an area of investigation not already receiving adequate or appropriate attention;
- It must demonstrate reasonable prospects for scientific growth and sufficient funding; and

- The proposed organizational changes should improve communication, management, priority setting, and accountability in terms of the nation's health care scientific endeavors.

Organized nursing was quick to describe the proposed national institute of nursing as meeting these criteria. Such an institute would focus on research and research training, not on the delivery of service. It would extend the purview of NIH beyond the current biomedical focus to include essential research on health promotion, short- and long-term care needs, and the care of individuals and families faced with acute and chronic illnesses and disability. The lack of stable funding for such research in the past provided clear evidence that the research area, though important, was not receiving appropriate, or even adequate, attention. Considering reasonable prospects for scientific growth and funding, the profession argued that with over 6,000 doctorally prepared nurses, 40 doctoral programs in nursing, and well-established national and regional research organizations, nationally and regionally, as well as a number of established journals, the prospects for growth were obvious. The increased amount of funds available—$11.4 million for research and research training, together with the $5 million in startup funds for such a structural entity that had been appropriated by Congress for fiscal year 1985—suggested that prospects existed for increased funding (Staff, 1984). As McBride (1987, p. 2) commented, "the placement of an institute of nursing in the NIH would greatly improve both communication about the largest health care profession to other disciplines and the flow of information about NIH priorities to nursing, and would ultimately bring nurses into the setting of national research priorities."

In 1985, both houses of Congress proposed bills similar to those vetoed earlier. In October 1985, Senate and House conferees resolved the differences regarding reauthorizing legislation for the NIH. A key feature in the new version of the bill as it emerged from the conference committee was a provision authorizing the NCNR within NIH, a compromise that was a concession to the White House's earlier and continuing objections to creating new institutes. This bill was vetoed on November 8, 1985, but the veto was overridden by the House on November 12, by a vote of 380 to 32, and by the Senate on November 20, by a vote of 89 to 7.

The successful legislative bid for creating the NCNR at NIH was initially the result of careful consideration and systematic study by nursing professionals and others of its structural options for creating an entity that would most effectively promote the scientific excellence of its growing body of nursing knowledge. The establishment of the Center was also the result of a second historical movement within the discipline, namely, the unification of the professional organizations, functioning with one goal and one voice to accomplish what was a basic concern to all: the enhancement and facilitation of nursing science within the rich interdisciplinary community of scholars at NIH in order to generate knowledge that could guide nursing practice and improve patient care.

MISSION OF NCNR
IN RELATIONSHIP TO MISSION OF NIH

The general purpose of the NCNR is "the conduct and support of, and dissemination of information respecting, basic and clinical nursing research, training, and other programs in patient care research" (Health Research Extension Act of 1985). Nursing research focuses on investigations related to the "diagnosis or treatment of human responses to actual or potential health problems" (Merritt, 1986). Such research involves scientific inquiry into basic and clinical biomedical and behavioral processes, as well as into nursing therapeutics or interventions that are effective in patient care. The conceptual and methodologic approaches are interdisciplinary, drawing from a number of fields. The ultimate goal of nursing science and research is the improvement of nursing practice in order to enhance prevention, promote recovery, and maintain health.

The broad mission of the NIH is to improve the health of the people of the United States by increasing our understanding of the processes underlying human health and by acquiring new knowledge to help prevent, detect, diagnose, and treat disease. This broad mission is consistent with the purpose and defining characteristics of nursing research as cited above; however, there are certain characteristics (e.g., the organization of programs around major diseases) that distinguish NIH's orientation from the orientations of nursing research. One project in the early 1980s (Stevenson, 1983) showed certain major nursing research topics were not in keeping with the mission and goals of the traditional NIH organizational entities. A number of proposals submitted for consideration to the institutes by nurse scientists did not fit the mission of individual bureaus, institutes, and divisions. These applications included substantive questions on, for example, (1) care processes, (2) communication as an intervention, and (3) the family as a health care target. The challenge of the next several years will be to bring these different types of research into a collaborative relationship with the traditional foci of NIH.

STRUCTURE AND PROGRAMS OF NCNR

NCNR Within NIH and HHS

The NCNR is one of a number of structural entities within NIH. Within the broader structure of the Department of Health and Human Services, NIH is only one organization within the Public Health Service; it is controlled by the Secretary of Health and Human Services through the Assistant Secretary of Health. Within NIH itself, there is the office of the director, a number of administrative offices that facilitate the scientific work of the extramural and intramural programs, and the individual bureaus, institutes, divisions, and centers, to which the NCNR is the newest addition.

Components of NCNR

The NCNR is made up of the office of the director; the professional nursing program staff, who are responsible for facilitating and enhancing the scientific efforts of the nursing community; and the administrative staff, who facilitate the conduct of program activities. The defined program areas, or "branches," are the major focal point of the NCNR's functions. Each of the three branches is administered by a branch chief, who is responsible to the director of extramural programs (DEP). The DEP is charged with overall coordination of the branches and is responsible to the director of the NCNR.

During the early steps leading to the authorization of the NCNR, the national definition of nursing research was refined and visibly marketed by the discipline. The guiding legislative statements were extracted from policy papers formulated and published by the professional bodies (Cabinet on Nursing Research, 1985; Sigma Theta Tau, 1986). Such policy statements had been motivated by requests from nursing leaders in the federal arena, such as Jo Eleanor Elliott, director of the Division of Nursing, where nursing research was located before the move to NIH. Elliott felt the need to begin setting a national research agenda for nursing, but wished to base the agenda on research priorities established by the discipline and its community of scholars. One of the documents (Cabinet on Nursing Research, 1985) emphasized the need for nurses to study health promotion and disease prevention in individuals and families, as well as the care of acutely or chronically ill, disabled, or dying persons and their families. These areas of scientific concern were directly reflected in the legislation authorizing the NCNR.

The legislatively stated general purpose of the NCNR is the "conduct and support of, and dissemination of information respecting, basic and clinical nursing research, training, and other programs in patient care research" (Health Research Extension Act of 1985). A subsequent section of the law suggests that the support and training programs can be established in the "study and investigation of the prevention of disease, health promotion, and the nursing care of individuals with and the families of individuals with acute and chronic illnesses." Patient care research may also address ethical and public policy concerns that will have a profound effect on the delivery of patient care. The program branches in the NCNR were structured to reflect the legislative mandate.

Health Promotion/Disease Prevention Branch. Research in the area of health promotion is designed to increase individuals' and their families' ability to resist illness or disability and maintain health throughout the lifespan. Health promotion research is not directed at any particular illness or disability but focuses on the health of the population. An example of a study to promote health would be the investigation of nutritional requirements across the various developmental phases of life.

Disease prevention research, on the other hand, includes studies that are applicable to intercepting the onset of an illness or disability. These investigations promote protection of individuals and families through the identification of biomedical, behavioral, and environmental factors that cause and prevent illness. In addition, disease prevention includes "the development or refinement of methods to enhance the abilities of individuals and families to respond to actual or potential health problems" (Merritt, 1986, p. 84).

Acute and Chronic Illness Branch. Research in this area deals broadly with "responses to acute and chronic illness and disability across the life span. It considers biomedical, behavioral, and environmental factors that contribute to the causes, prevalence, amelioration, and remediation of illness and disability" (Merritt, 1986, p. 84). Examples include basic and clinical studies in the biomedical and behavioral processes and therapeutics of acute and chronic illness.

Nursing Systems and Special Programs Branch. Investigations in nursing systems address the environmental factors that influence the effective and efficient delivery of care to clients and their patients. Merritt (1986, p. 85) cited several examples: "comparisons of the outcomes of home care, long-term care and/or hospital care; identifying the mechanisms responsible for different outcomes; research in methods to improve the delivery of nursing care in underserved areas; and studies of innovative approaches to the delivery and cost of nursing care in various types of agencies." One special program emphasis involves ethical issues related to patient care and patient care research, e.g., the ethical processes and dilemmas underlying clincial decisions required of patients, family members, and health care providers on questions such as death and dying, transplantation, and prolongation of life.

Research Training Program. Research training and career development cuts across all three branches of the NCNR. The responsibility of this transbranch area is to ensure the existence of an adequate cadre of well-trained nurse scientists to meet the nursing research needs of the future. Staff organize and facilitate, with the Nursing Science Review Committee, the initial scientific and technical merit review of the National Research Service Award (NRSA) training program for individual and institutional predoctoral and postdoctoral fellowships and career development awards. Several new NCNR directions in research training and career development have been initiated in 1987. These include a new emphasis on the NRSA institutional awards and the introduction of career development awards, such as the Academic and Clinical Investigator Awards. Senior fellowship awards have also been offered.

National Advisory Council.   An NCNR Advisory Council (NCNRAC) of 17 members has been chartered. As mandated by the legislation, the membership includes nurse scientists (58 percent of the voting members), consumers of nursing care, physicians, epidemiologists, and corporate and hospital administrators, as well as several ex officio members (the Deputy Surgeon General, the director of the Division of Nursing of the Health Resources and Services Agency, the VA chief of nursing research, and a representative of the office of the Assistant Secretary of Defense for Health Affairs). The Council is responsible for providing consultation and advice on policies, programs, and future initiatives to the director of the NCNR.

Staff, Physical Space, and Budget.   Six professional scientists and three support workers moved to NIH with the research programs from the Division of Nursing at the Bureau of Health Professions with the HRSA. The number of full-time equivalent (FTE) staff members has been increased from these original nine to a current total of 28 (seven positions remain to be filled). As would be expected, space is a problem. The NCNR staff is located in two sets of temporary quarters until the permanent area is renovated. A permanent space for the NCNR is being prepared in the major administrative building on the NIH Bethesda campus, which houses the director's offices and sections of the other institutes and divisions.

The NCNR budget has increased from the $11,296,000 available in 1985 to $19,000,000. For the first time in a number of years, the President's 1988 budget allocated monies for nursing research as a line item. The move of nursing research to NIH has, to date, increased the amount and stability of resources underlying the discipline's scientific programs.

FUTURE INITIATIVES FOR NCNR

Incorporating the concept of nursing research into the mainstream with other health care sciences necessitates a series of future initiatives. These initiatives have been shared and discussed with the members of the NCNRAC.

National Nursing Research Agenda

One of the first initiatives for the NCNR will be the development of a National Nursing Research Agenda to articulate the nursing research priorities of the center to the nursing scientific community and to guide the allocation of resources. Therefore, the creation of a five-year plan and an annual review of the program priorities to guide funding decisions is required of all NIH Institutes. The NCNR staff, in collaboration with the members of the National Advisory Council and members of the nursing scientific community, is developing such an agenda, which articulates the scientific priorities of our discipline.

A number of statements delineating nursing research priorities have been published since 1983 by our profession's major organizations (Cabinet on Nursing Research, 1985; Sigma Theta Tau, 1986; American Association of Colleges of Nursing, 1981; Lewandowski & Hositsky, 1983; Oberst, 1978; American Organization of Nurse Executives, 1986). These priority statements and others will be analyzed and synthesized in an effort to create a consensus statement of priorities within our discipline. Such a statement will then be presented for consideration to the members of the scientific community as well as to members of the National Advisory Council. The National Nursing Research Agenda will be formulated from the ensuing deliberations.

Although the five-year plan will be guided by the National Nursing Research Agenda, it will also reflect various alternatives for funding awards. In addition to the traditional type of individual investigator award (RO1), increasing use may be made of program awards, the First Independent Research Support and Transition Awards (FIRST), multisite research support, longer-term research support, Method to Extend Research in Time (MERIT) awards, and Center awards. We hope to extend a number of traditional NIH award mechanisms to the nursing scientific community.

Series of Research Training Awards

A second inititative that has been initiated at the NCNR is the increased encouragement of nurse scientists to take advantage of a series of research training and career development awards. A number of different alternatives for scientific training opportunities have already become available to nurse researchers in the last 12 to 18 months through the Clinical Investigator Award and the Academic Investigator Award.

Traditionally, the nursing discipline has made excellent use of predoctoral and, to a more limited extent, postdoctoral NRSA fellowship awards. The limited use of the NRSA Institutional Research Training awards has been expanded to increase the number of students studying within a larger cadre of fellows and a critical mass of faculty scientists. Although no senior fellowships have been offered to date, this program is also available to seasoned researchers who wish to further their investigations in a specific field of research with other colleagues in similar scientific endeavors.

It is hoped that nurse researchers will think of research training as an ongoing, integral part of their scientific careers rather than as a one-time fellowship to complete basic predoctoral study. For example, in the basic and biomedical disciplines, postdoctoral study is a traditional follow-through to predoctoral education. Postdoctoral education is now being increasingly considered by nursing scientists as well. In addition to the predoctoral/postdoctoral training opportunities, it is possible for our scientists to work in educational or clinical health care agencies for several years and then to return for either an Academic or a Clinical Investigator Award, which allows them to work with an individual in their scientific field who has had more experience. A senior fellowship allows individuals who may be serving as mentors to postdoctoral clinical investigators or academic investigators to return for further research and stimulation in their own area of expertise. Thus, a wide array of research training and career development awards are available for use by our scientists, providing ongoing intellectual stimulation and revitalization.

Increased Collaboration with Other Disciplines

One of the major reasons for moving nursing research to NIH was to further formal and informal networking with other health care sciences. A number of opportunities exist for increasing collaboration with other discipliens. Several strategies were used by the research staff when they were at the Division of Nursing, and these have been continued and extended with the creation of the NCNR at NIH for cofunding of shared areas of research (e.g., incontinence in the elderly).

Postdoctoral awards are available for nurse scientists who wish to study with investigators in other disciplines. They allow the nurse researcher to function as an investigative member of a scientific team while being supported by NCNR nursing funds. The NIH Task Force on Nursing Research (1984) suggested other mechanisms for increased collaboration, such as appointment of nurse scientists to the study panels and advisory councils for other NIH institutes, along with provision for research training, as discussed earlier.

Intramural Research Programs

One of the major initiatives the NCNR staff will take in the next several years will be the development and operation of an intramural research program that is active both at the Clinical Center and within other agencies. Traditionally, the intramural research programs within NIH structural units have been based primarily in the Clinical Center or in general clinical centers supported throughout the country. Most certainly, nursing will need a collaborative intramural program within this framework. Strategies will be considered whereby patients can be contacted and enrolled for participation in nursing research investigations.

The National Center may also wish to consider an intramural program that is partially "without walls." Since nursing research includes studies conducted in a number of health care agencies of diverse types and structures, the NCNR staff ought to consider the creation of intramural sites within home health care agencies, public health agencies, nursing homes, community hospitals, and other settings. This would facilitate investigations that must be conducted in specific types of agencies, as well as investigations that study the movement of and outcomes for clients as they are discharged from one kind of care and admitted to another across a variety of agencies.

The possibilities for the intramural research programs appear to be numerous. It will be exciting for the staff to develop such program initiatives in collaboration with members of the scientific community.

International Program

Dr. Faye Abdellah (1987), as a member of the National Advisory Council, has been particularly helpful in considering a possible international initiative for the National Center. Access to multiple populations from diverse cultures would allow the generation and testing of nursing knowledge within a rich context.

The operationalization of these initiatives will be outlined in the National Center's five-year plan, which will basically be guided by the nursing research priorities identified in the National Nursing Research Agenda. Such a plan will also delineate the resources required to implement these initiatives, along with the research support and research training mechanisms that will be needed for its success.

CONCLUSION

In summary, moving nursing research to NIH was the result of the profession's commitment and unified posture towards a common goal. Nurses, as clinicians, educators, executives, and scientists, agreed on a common issue: the need to place the discipline's science in the arena with other health care research in order to enhance the excellence and rich interdisciplinary nature of both the evolving body of nursing science and its contribution to the improvement of health care in this country.

This past year has witnessed the implementation of the NCNR within NIH. This move has entailed the expenditure of many hours on planning the program, structure, and policies; outlining new staff positions; becoming oriented to the NIH procedure; opening to nursing many traditional NIH award systems; employing new and different types of staff; establishing new grants management procedures; and chartering and activating the National Advisory Council, to name only a few of the numerous endeavors.

The challenges of the future are evident in the initiative statements. Moving nursing research to NIH has provided a national focal point for scientific activity in this country, as the IOM (1983) recommended a few years ago. Nurses and nurse scientists can be expected to continue to capitalize on this opportunity.

REFERENCES

Abdellah, F. G. (1987). Remarks to the National Advisory Council, National Center for Nursing Research, NIH, June 1987.

American Association of Colleges of Nursing. (1981). Nursing research: Position statement. Washington, DC: Author.

American Organization of Nurse Executives. (1986). Final report of the ad hoc committee on nursing administration research. Chicago: Author.

Cabinet on Nursing Research. (1985). *Directions for nursing research: Toward the twenty-first century.* Kansas City, MO: American Nurses' Association.

Institute of Medicine. (1983). *Nursing and nursing education: Public policies and private actions.* Washington, DC: National Academy Press.

Institute of Medicine. (1984). *Responding to health needs and scientific opportunity: The organizational structure of the National Institutes of Health.* Washington, DC: National Academy Press.

Lewandowski, L. A., & Hositsky, A. M. (1983). Research priorities for critical care nursing: A study by the American Association of Critical-Care Nurses. *Heart & Lung, 12*(1), 35–44.

McBride, A. B. (1987). The National Center for Nursing Research, National Institutes of Health. *Social Policy Report, 2*(2), 1–11.

Merritt, D. H. (1986). The National Center for Nursing Research. *Image, 18*(3), 84–85.

National Institutes of Health Task Force on Nursing Research. (1984, Dec.). *Report to the Director 1984.* Bethesda, MD: Author.

Oberst, M. T. (1978). Priorities in cancer nursing research. *Cancer Nursing, 1,* 281–290.

Sigma Theta Tau. (1986). *Ten-year plan for knowledge: Development, dissemination, utilization.* Indianapolis: Author.

Staff. (1984, October 12). Continuing resolution increases funding for nursing education and research. *Legislative Network for Nurses.*

Stevenson, J. (1983). *New investigator federal sector grantsmanship project: Final report.* Kansas City, MO: American Nurses' Association.

ACKNOWLEDGMENT

The staff of the NCNR contributed to the program information incorporated into this paper.

THE NURSING MINIMUM DATA SET: BENEFITS AND IMPLICATIONS

Harriet H. Werley, PhD, RN
Distinguished Professor
School of Nursing
University of Wisconsin-Milwaukee

CeCelia R. Zorn, MSN, RN
Doctoral Student and Project Assistant
School of Nursing
University of Wisconsin-Milwaukee

The Nursing Minimum Data Set (NMDS) is an initial effort to establish uniform standards for the collection of the minimum essential nursing data. It draws on the documentation of the nursing process that occurs whenever nurses provide care to people in any setting. This establishment of uniform standards is crucial in the changing clinical scene as the dawn of the 21st century approaches.

There are a variety of factors that are influencing all of nursing practice at an unprecedented pace. Nurses are practicing in more diverse settings than ever before. The move in health care from acute care settings to community settings is changing the employment practices of many nurses, especially those who graduated two or three years ago. With the movement to more autonomous practice comes a need for nurses to accept increased accountability —accountability not only for the use of resources but also for specific interventions to achieve a desired client outcome.

The growth in the aging population and the increasing cost of health care are also exerting far-reaching effects. The increase in the elderly population in the United States is probably the most dramatic change in the 20th century. According to the 1980 census, one person in nine is over 65 years old today, whereas only one in 25 was in 1900. On the basis of projected growth between 1976 and 2000, it is estimated that the 65- to 74-year-old age group will increase

105

by 23 percent, the 75- to 84-year-old group by 57 percent, and the 85 and over group by 11 percent (Rich & Baum, 1984). With the growing elderly population, there also is an increase in chronic diseases and accompanying socioeconomic issues that must be addressed. Closely related to the increase in the elderly population are rapidly rising health care expenditures. In 1981, health care costs totaled $1,223 per person and accounted for 9.8 percent of the gross national product. For Medicare alone, the costs were estimated to be $57 billion in 1983, and were projected to rise to $112 billion by 1988 (Barger, 1985).

As the minimum data set is established for nursing in the changing health care arena, its development must be geared to the entire nursing profession: a data set that is setting-specific would serve only that area of nursing practice, and it might result in division of nurses by health care settings. A minimum data set applicable to all of nursing would facilitate the establishment and use of a common language, as it were, which is needed by the profession and by others in the health care field. Within this new environment of increased acceptance of accountability by nurses, changes in practice settings, increases in cost of health care, and the growth of the elderly population—along with an existing and projected shortage of professional nurses—the NMDS will be explored as a link in the integration of computers into nursing care across all practice settings.

DERIVATION, CONCEPT, AND PURPOSES
OF THE NMDS

Uniform Minimum Health Data Sets

A Uniform Minimum Health Data Set (UMHDS) has been defined as "a minimum set of items of information with uniform definitions and categories, concerning a specific aspect or dimension of the health care system which meets the essential needs of multiple data users" (Health Information Policy Council [HIPC], 1983, p. 3). The key phrase is "multiple data users"; it is not only nurses who are involved. The concept, adopted first in 1972, was used in earlier efforts to develop national health data standards and guidelines (Murnaghan & White, 1970). Of the patient- or client-focused UMHDSs developed previously, which are concerned with long-term care, hospital discharge, and ambulatory care (National Committee on Vital and Health Statistics [NCVHS], 1980a, 1980b, 1981), the Uniform Hospital Discharge Data Set (UHDDS) is the one in widespread use today (HIPC, 1983, 1984, 1985).

Concept of the NMDS

The NMDS is built on the concept of the UMHDS. It represents the first attempt to standardize the collection of essential nursing data. By adapting the definition of a UMHDS, the NMDS can be defined as a minimum set of items of information with uniform definitions and categories concerning the specific dimension of nursing that meets the information needs of multiple data users in the health care system. The NMDS would include those specific items of information that are used on a regular basis by the majority of nurses across all types of settings in the delivery of care.

Purposes of the NMDS

The purposes of the NMDS are (1) to establish comparability of nursing data across clinical populations, settings, geographic areas, and time; (2) to describe the nursing care of patients or clients and their families in a variety of settings, both institutional and noninstitutional; (3) to demonstrate or project trends regarding nursing care needs and allocation of nursing resources to patients or clients according to their health problems or nursing diagnoses; and (4) to stimulate nursing research through links to the detailed data existing in nursing information systems (NISs) and other health-care information systems (HCISs).

CONSENSUAL IDENTIFICATION OF THE NMDS

Follow-Through on Earlier Work

The current project, the aim of which is to identify the NMDS, is in essence a follow-through on some of Werley's earlier work, which was done at the University of Illinois College of Nursing. During that time Werley served on the Health Care Technology Study Section of the National Center for Health Services Research and was involved in reviewing research proposals for many of the medical and hospital information systems that are now large and well recognized. Out of concern that nurses were not sufficiently active in the development of information systems in the health fields, she and a colleague developed and conducted a Nursing Information Systems Conference at the University of Illinois, Chicago, in 1977. In that conference, an effort was made to stimulate nurses to move toward computerization of nursing data and submission of proposals to develop NISs; in addition, one of the small work groups was given the problem of identifying a basic nursing data set (see Figure 1). The group did well, as Newcomb (1981) documents, especially considering the short time that could be allotted for group work in that particular conference. Apparently, however, the timing was not right for nursing, and no one seemed to fo" w through on the idea of identifying and developing a basic nursing data set. Shortly after Werley moved to the University of Wisconsin–Milwaukee in 1983, she concluded that the time was right, opened the subject again, and assembled a small group to work with her on this idea.

Figure 1. Categories of a Basic Nursing Data Set

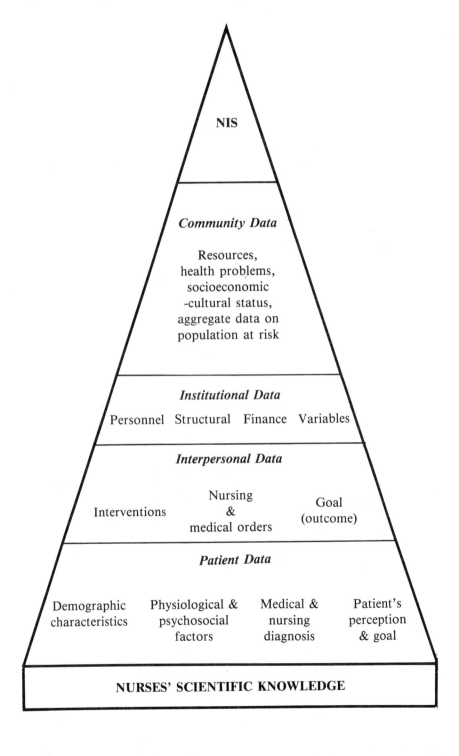

Efforts at the University of Wisconsin–Milwaukee

Subsequent development occurred at the three-day invitational NMDS Conference held in Wisconsin in 1985, which was sponsored by the University of Wisconsin–Milwaukee School of Nursing and funded largely by the Hospital Corporation of America Foundation (Werley & Lang, in press; Werley, Lang, & Westlake, 1986a, 1986b). The participants at this conference included nurse experts in a variety of areas; health policy spokespersons; information systems, health data, and health records specialists; and persons knowledgeable about development of the UMHDSs. The 65 conference participants were assigned to one of six task forces, each of which was directed to identify the elements of a particular category of the nursing process (nursing assessment, nursing diagnoses, nursing interventions, nursing outcomes, nursing intensity, or demographics). The task forces also were asked to define their identified elements and, where time permitted, to identify measures or subelements. A postconference task force reviewed and refined the data set developed by the conference task forces.

Data Set Elements

The NMDS includes three broad categories of elements: (1) nursing care, (2) patient or client demographics, and (3) service elements (see Table 1). Elements that also are included in the previously mentioned UHDDS (HIPC, 1985; NCVHS, 1980b) are indicated by an asterisk in Table 1. Elements comparable to those already being collected need not be recollected in hospitals, when they can be obtained through existing relational data-base management systems.

Nursing intervention was included in the NMDS during the pilot testing period so that the feasibility of adding it as an element could be assessed. Before this element can be recommended fully, there must be an acceptable, exhaustive, and mutually exclusive coding scheme for categorizing nursing interventions. It is urgent that further research and development be done on a classification scheme for interventions. Bulechek, drawing on earlier work on interventions (Bulechek & McCloskey, 1985), has assembled a team to address this matter, and there also are plans to have an American Nurses' Association group work on development of an intervention taxonomy.

PILOT TESTING RESULTS

The pilot test of the NMDS, directed by Dr. Elizabeth C. Devine, included the records of 116 subjects from four types of clinical sites: a hospital, a nursing home, a home health care agency, and two clinics affiliated with a teaching hospital. Overall intercoder agreement was a satisfactory 91 percent,

Table 1.   Elements of the Nursing Minimum Data Set

Nursing care elements
Nursing diagnosis
Nursing intervention
Nursing outcome
Intensity of nursing care

Patient or client demographic elements
Personal identification*
Date of birth*
Sex*
Race and ethnicity*
Residence*

Service elements
Unique facility or service agency number*
Unique health record number of patient or client
Unique number of principal registered nurse provider
Episode admission or encounter date*
Discharge or termination date*
Disposition of patient or client*
Expected payer for most of this bill
        (anticipated financial guarantor for services)*

*Elements included in the UHDDS.

with an item-specific range of 57 to 100 percent. The implication of these results is that the definitions and protocol for coding were generally acceptable, although a few elements need refinement. Most of the NMDS elements were available for more than 90 percent of the cases. The exceptions were unique number of principal registered nurse provider, which was never available; ethnicity, which was available only 9 percent of the time; race, which was available for 71 percent of the subjects; resolution status, which was available for 79 percent of the documented nursing diagnoses; and personal identification number of the client, which was available for 86 percent of the subjects. A conclusion that can be drawn from these results is that existing records were an adequate source for most of the elements in the NMDS. More details about the NMDS pilot testing are available elsewhere (Devine & Werley, 1987).

PERCEIVED BENEFITS AND IMPLICATIONS

The benefits of the NMDS for nurses and nursing are highlighted, since nurses need to work toward building a system capable of ongoing collection of nursing's essential data. If the NMDS were adopted nationwide with a system of ongoing data collection, the following benefits could be expected:

1. Access to comparable minimum nursing care and resources data on local, regional, and national levels;
2. Enhanced documentation of nursing care provided;
3. Identification of trends related to client problems and nursing care provided;
4. Impetus to improve costing of nursing services;
5. Improved data for quality assurance evaluations;
6. Impetus to develop and refine nursing information systems;
7. Comparative research on nursing care, including research on nursing diagnosis, nursing interventions, resolution status of client problems, and referral for further nursing services; and
8. Contributions toward advancing nursing as a research-based discipline.

The specific implications of the NMDS for nurse researchers, nurse educators, and clinical nurses will be presented in the immediately following chapters. The remainder of the present chapter is devoted to general comments on the status of the NMDS project and a brief enumeration of future directions for the NMDS.

STATUS OF THE NMDS PROJECT

The NMDS was reviewed by the Health Information Policy Council of the U. S. Department of Health and Human Services. After a positive response from the HIPC, the Assistant Secretary for Health requested that the National Committee on Vital and Health Statistics conduct a detailed review of the NMDS and report its recommendations to him by January 1987. The NCVHS is the civilian consultant group that advises the Assistant Secretary for Health on matters of health statistics, including uniform minimum health data sets. To facilitate this review, Werley was invited to present and discuss the work done on the NMDS with members of the NCVHS in October 1986. Devine accompanied her to Washington, DC, for this meeting and participated in the discussion.

In essence, the content of the NCVHS recommendations and a letter from the Assistant Secretary for Health adhered to the view that the NMDS holds promise for a range of research uses, and that these research uses probably are best met through targeted research efforts. The NCVHS members also identified several areas of the proposed data where additional research and development are needed (e.g., nursing diagnosis and intensity of care). In addition, the NCVHS expressed concern about the desirability of a profession-specific uniform minimum data set, as opposed to a setting-based one. We were urged to explore interest and funding support from several U.S. Department of Health and Human Services Units, among them the National Institutes of Health National Center for Nursing Research, which was considered likely to support work on interventions and procedures.

A research proposal is now being developed that requests external funds to conduct a field study of the NMDS, using a larger number of health care facilities of various types to study the availability and reliability of the data. Building on the results of the pilot testing, efforts also will be made to demonstrate the types of research that can be done through use of the NMDS alone, as well as through use of the NMDS plus data obtained through data audit trails to the health records or computerized information systems at the institutional level. Initially, this proposal was to have been ready before the February 1, 1987, deadline, but this proved impossible, because of a cut in resources at the very time when the workload on the NMDS project was excessive. Efforts are continually being made to disseminate word about the NMDS, and the benefits and implications for nurses and nursing are discussed at both national and international meetings. The implications of the NMDS for the health care industry and the setting of health policy are also highlighted as deemed appropriate.

FUTURE DIRECTIONS FOR THE NMDS

Without going into detail about future directions, we believe that the following are the essential tasks that this project must perform in the near future:

1. To conduct a field study of the NMDS with a larger sample of the four different types of health care settings;

2. To demonstrate the types of research that can be done with the NMDS elements alone, as well as with the NMDS expanded through the use of data audit trails to additional data in the NIS or HCIS at the facility level;

3. To conduct a national field study of the NMDS;

4. To plan for local, regional, and national sessions on nursing documentation per the nursing process and the NMDS definitions, in order to promote comparable data;

5. To encourage computerization of NISs nationwide, so as to facilitate data audit trails from the NMDS to the more detailed raw data in NISs, HCISs, or health records for research purposes; and

6. To stimulate interest in and facilitate accomplishment of Resolution 24 on computerization of nursing services data, which was passed by the American Nurses' Association House of Delegates at the 1986 convention.

Computerization of nursing services data should be one of nursing's top priorities, for in this information age nursing cannot support its stands on many matters that have health policy implications unless it has appropriate, retrievable data. Too frequently today, health policy is set on the basis of incomplete data, for the nursing data are not there. What will nursing do about this? Are nursing service directors, or vice presidents for nursing, seeing to it that they get nursing's fair share of the total dollars spent on their facility for computerization? To bring nursing up to date in the age of information takes more than lip service: it requires immediate action on the part of leaders in nursing services.

REFERENCES

Barger, S. E. (1985). Nursing centers: Here today, gone tomorrow. In J. C. McCloskey & H. K. Grace (Eds.), *Current issues in nursing* (2nd ed.) (pp. 752–760). Boston: Blackwell.

Bulechek, G. M., & McClosky, J. C. (1985). *Nursing interventions: Treatments for nursing diagnoses.* Philadelphia: W. B. Saunders.

Devine, E. C., & Werley, H. H. (1987). *Test of the Nursing Minimum Data Set: Availability of data and reliability.* Manuscript submitted for publication.

Health Information Policy Council. (1983). *Background paper: Uniform minimum health data sets.* Unpublished manuscript, U.S. Department of Health and Human Services, Washington, DC.

Health Information Policy Council. (1984). *1984 Revision of the uniform hospital discharge data set.* Unpublished manuscript, U. S. Department of Health and Human Services, Washington, DC.

Health Information Policy Council. (1983, July 31). 1984 Revision of the uniform hospital discharge data set. *Federal Register, 50*(147), 31038–31040.

Murnaghan, J. H. & White, K. L. (Eds.). (1970). Hospital discharge data: Report of the Conference on Hospital Discharge Abstract Systems. *Medical Care, 8*(4, Suppl.), 1–215.

National Committee on Vital and Health Statistics. (1980a). *Long-term health care: Minimum data set* (DHHS Publication No. PHS 80-1158). Hyattsville, MD: U. S. Department of Health and Human Services, National Center for Health Statistics.

National Committee on Vital and Health Statistics. (1980b). *Uniform hospital discharge data: Minimum data set* (DHEW Publication No. PHS 80-1157). Hyattsville, MD: U.S. Department of Health, Education, and Welfare, National Center for Health Statistics.

National Committee on Vital and Health Statistics. (1981). *Uniform ambulatory medical care: Minimum data set* (DHHS Publication No. 81-1161). Hyattsville, MD: U.S. Department of Health and Human Services, National Center for Health Statistics.

Newcomb, B. J. (1981). Issues related to identifying and systematizing data—group discussions. In H. H. Werley & M. R. Grier (Eds.), *Nursing information systems.* New York: Springer.

Rich, B. M., & Baum, R. (1984). *The aging: A guide to public policy.* Pittsburgh, PA: University of Pittsburgh Press.

Werley, H. H., & Grier, M. R. (Eds.). (1981). *Nursing information systems.* New York: Springer.

Werley, H. H., & Lang, N. M. (Eds.) (in press). *Identification of the nursing minimum data set.* New York: Springer.

Werley, H. H., Lang, N. M., & Westlake, S. K. (1986a). Brief summary of the Nursing Minimum Data Set Conference. *Nursing Management, 17*(7), 42–45.

Werley, H. H., Lang, N. M., & Westlake, S. K. (1986b). The Nursing Minimum Data Set Conference: Executive summary. *Journal of Professional Nursing, 2,* 117–224.

ACKNOWLEDGMENT

The Blanhe Foundation provided partial support for the writing of this paper.

THE NURSING MINIMUM DATA SET: BENEFITS AND IMPLICATIONS FOR NURSE RESEARCHERS

Elizabeth C. Devine, PhD, RN
Assistant Professor
School of Nursing
University of Wisconsin–Milwaukee

Before the various benefits and implications of the Nursing Minimum Data Set (NMDS) for nurse researchers are enumerated, it is important to set the record straight: the NMDS is *not* a panacea for nursing research. As with any single entity, its impact is somewhat limited in scope. One can easily imagine areas of nursing research that will not be influenced in any way by the widespread adoption of the NMDS. These areas include many kinds of historical research, qualitative research, and methodologic research, to name a few

If, however, one's research interests are focused within the broad areas of the process, outcome, or cost of nursing care, then widespread adoption of the NMDS may yield data that are invaluable. It is also important to remember that since the intention is to collect NMDS data in all settings where nurses regularly provide care, this data resource would not be limited to specific regions of the country or to a narrow range of clinical nursing problems.

There are basically three ways in which NMDS could benefit nursing research: (1) the data could be all that is needed for research; (2) they could provide the basis for an audit trail; or (3) they could provide the basis for a sampling frame. The "stand-alone use" of the NMDS involves basing an entire study on data contained within the NMDS. The "audit trail use" involves employing the NMDS as a basis for an audit trail back to the more detailed nursing information system (NIS) or the health information system at the facility level. In this second approach, the NMDS data could be supplemented with other data from the health record, which would then provide all the data needed for a particular study. Finally, the "sampling frame use" involves concurrent or retrospective review of NMDS data to provide the basis for establishing a sampling frame for research based entirely, or primarily, on non-NMDS data.

115

POSSIBLE RESEARCH USES OF NMDS

When research projects based on the three uses of the NMDS identified above are being considered, it is essential to keep in mind the assumptions underlying widespread adoption of the NMDS. It is assumed that if the NMDS is adopted, all of the NMDS elements identified elsewhere in this volume (p. 105) by Werley and Zorn would be collected, that the scope of data collection would involve all patients or clients, and that NMDS data would be collected in all settings where nurses routinely provide care.

Stand-Alone Use

The following are examples of some research that could be based on use of the NMDS alone:

1. Describing the nursing interventions used for selected nursing diagnoses;
2. Describing the resolution status of specific nursing diagnoses and the incidence of referrals for further nursing care after discharge;
3. Comparing the staffing patterns and hours of nursing care for patients with selected nursing diagnoses in specific types of settings—locally, regionally, and nationally;
4. Describing the age, gender, and expected payor of patients with selected nursing diagnoses, who are or are not referred for further nursing care after discharge from the hospital;
5. Comparing the intensity of nursing care provided to patients with selected nursing diagnoses in different health care settings—hospitals, nursing homes, home health care agencies, and ambulatory care;
6. Comparing length of hospital stay for patients with specific nursing diagnoses—locally, regionally, and nationally; and
7. Describing the resolution status of selected nursing diagnoses according to various staffing patterns;

Audit Trail Use

The research one could do if the NMDS was used to facilitate an audit trail back to the existing health record includes the following possibilities:

1. Comparing the intensity of nursing care for selected medical diagnoses in different health care settings—hospitals, nursing homes, home health care agencies, and ambulatory care;
2. Comparing the staff mix hours of nursing care, or both, for selected medical diagnoses in specific types of settings—locally, regionally, and nationally;

3. Describing the number and type of pharmaceutical agents prescribed for patients with selected nursing or medical diagnoses and their relationship to nursing home placement;

4. Comparing the use pattern of ancillary services (e.g., postoperative respiratory therapy) for patients with selected medical or nursing diagnoses across settings; and

5. Describing the urinary continence status at admission to the acute-care setting of patients with selected medical or nursing diagnoses and its relationship to nursing home placement after discharge from the hospital.

Sampling Frame Use

Finally, the NMDS might also be used to identify a sampling frame for research, based primarily or entirely on non-NMDS data. With this approach, one could identify the following:

1. Patients with a specific nursing diagnosis;

2. Institutions or clinical units with various staffing patterns;

3. Patients who have been referred for further nursing care after discharge;

4. Patients with selected nursing diagnoses that have been treated with specific nursing interventions;

5. Patients with specific nursing diagnoses that are unresolved at discharge; and

6. Patients with specific nursing diagnoses that had particularly long or short hospital stays.

PREREQUISITES

All these potential research uses of the NMDS data that presumably will benefit nurse researchers depend on certain prerequisites that nurse researchers, administrators, and educators can help address. First and foremost, various data elements, such as nursing diagnoses, nursing interventions, and intensity of nursing care, must be refined and validated through basic research. This is essential if we are to have confidence in the nursing data that are collected. Second, nursing data must be recorded more consistently and saved, so that the data will in fact be retrievable from the health record. The NMDS is based on record review, and if the data are not recorded and saved, it cannot be implemented. Administrators and clinicians will have the most impact here, but researchers can contribute by being involved in the development and testing of computerized information systems. Third, those who see the benefit in having these data available on a local, regional, and national basis must take action to ensure that the NMDS will become a reality. Individual clinicians, administrators, and educators can help by encouraging documentation that follows the nursing process and that enables specific interventions and outcomes to be linked with nursing diagnoses. Researchers can encourage adoption of the NMDS by conducting high-quality research that demonstrates the valuable information that can be obtained through large-scale studies based on the NMDS.

CONCLUSION

The road from conception of the NMDS to federally mandated adoption of it is a long one. Valid and reliable nursing data, available for all clients from a wide range of nursing practice settings, would be an incredible resource for nurse researchers. If that resource is to be become a reality, clinicians, administrators, educators, and researchers must collaborate and mobilize the resources needed to make it one.

THE NURSING MINIMUM DATA SET:
BENEFITS AND IMPLICATIONS FOR NURSE EDUCATORS

Joanne Comi McCloskey, PhD, RN
Professor and Chair
Organizations and Systems
University of Iowa

The achievement of a nursing minimum data set (NMDS) would provide standardized data describing nursing practice that could be used for multiple purposes. The aim of this paper is to examine those purposes that are related to education.

The NMDS facilitates the collection of comparable clinical nursing data across populations, settings, regions, and time. Ideally, all health care institutions would collect health information on a computer, and each institution would summarize the relevant nursing information in a clinical nursing abstract, from which would be further abstracted the NMDS in an identical form for all institutions. The NMDS would provide direction for nursing information systems (NISs), which are still in their infancy. As Zielstorff (1984) and others have pointed out, the major impediment to the development of computerized NISs is the deficiencies in nursing's knowledge base:

> Those who work in the design and development of nursing information systems constantly bemoan the fact that there are so few clinical problems in nursing for which the etiology symptoms, treatment, and expected outcomes are known. There are no known probability estimates for prevalence or incidence of common nursing problems; or for relating symptoms to diagnosis, or treatment to outcome. Indeed, there is neither a standard terminology nor a widely accepted format for data gathering. It is impossible to derive hard and fast rules for computer assistance in decision making with such an ill-defined data base. (p. 9)

The minimum nursing data set provides a way of collecting nursing knowledge that would lead to the development of better NISs, which in turn would modify what we collect to construct the NMDS.

FUTURE OF NMDS IN NURSING EDUCATION

In the future, the NMDS could be required for third-party reimbursement, and the clinical nursing abstract could be required for accreditation. If an institution had to submit standardized data in order to get reimbursement or accreditation, it would create a mechanism to facilitate this. It would thus have increased interest in NISs, and the use of NISs would result not only in the NMDS but in large sets of data at the individual institutional level. Besides the elements of the nursing minimum data set, the clinical nursing abstracts would include assessment data, medical diagnoses, treatment data, financial data, and anything else an institution thought important. These data sets (the NMDS and the clinical nursing abstracts), if collected in a systematic way and computerized, have the potential (with help from nursing researchers) to revolutionize nursing education. They may revolutionize both the content and the process of nursing education—i.e., what we teach and how we teach.

Underlying the implementation of the minimum data set are several assumptions:

1. That all facilities or practices will document their services by means of a computer;
2. That the lists of nursing diagnoses, interventions, and outcomes used by the NMDS reflect current practice; and
3. That there are mechanisms in place to update the lists as practice changes.

Two main assumptions underly estimates of the uses and benefits of the NMDS in nursing education:

1. That nursing students have easy access to computers and are computer-literate; and
2. That schools of nursing education have access to data bases generated by practice settings.

None of these assumptions are really certainties. In fact, most of the assumptions and the implications for education remain to be evaluated. Their implementation will require many tough decisions en route.

My vision for the future of nursing education is that the NMDS and its institutional counterpart, the clinical nursing abstract, will become the source of nursing knowledge and will be used interactively to teach students clinical decision making. Once these data sets are collected, analyzed, and organized, they will be used to generate the practice-based knowledge that we will teach our beginning nurses. Students will be taught nursing content through actual client data rather than through textbook examples. Schools of nursing can access the data bases gathered by their colleagues in practice and use them in teaching. For example, a data base on the diagnosis "ineffective individual coping" can be accessed, and the student can study the associated interventions and outcomes and find out in what populations certain interventions are most effective for this diagnosis. They can access the assessment data for a particular group of patients and examine the etiologies, signs, symptoms, related medical diagnoses, and medical therapies recorded.

This may not seem to be a revolutionary development, but it is in sharp contrast with what we do now, which is to teach from medical-surgical textbooks, based mostly on medical knowledge; from nursing process books, based mostly on untested nursing theory; and from audiocassettes, films, and skills manuals, based mostly on tradition. We have students practice technical skills in a lab before they try them with patients, but at present they have little opportunity to practice the more difficult decision-making skills. In response to this situation, there has been a recent flush of books with case studies and some computer patient simulations. These are helpful, but they are clearly obsolescent when compared with an accessible interactive data base on diagnoses, etiologies, signs and symptoms, interventions and outcomes. This is not to say that future nursing education will use no books, films, lectures, or seminars; but rather that the data generated from systematic collection of nursing diagnoses, interventions, and outcomes will become the sources for textbook and classroom presentations. Nursing diagnosis and intervention textbooks based on tested theory will eventually replace our medical-surgical, pediatric, psychologic, and other textbooks, and we will see more films and audiocassettes demonstrating independent nursing interventions.

CHALLENGES

Nursing education is in for a rough stretch in the coming decade. There are three major challenges that nurse educators face, one in each of the three key areas—students, faculty, and curricula. In each area, I will outline the major challenge as I see it and then identify ways in which the NMDS can assist educators to meet the challenge.

Students

It has recently become well known, at least within nursing circles, that our enrollments are down. This problem is compounded by the shortage of nurses in the practice setting. The challenge to nurse educators is determining how to maintain both a sufficient quantity and a high quality of students. But what is sufficient? Can both quantity and quality be ensured? What additional resources and methods do we need? Some of the new potential pools of students need more remediation than in the past. The answer preferred by many faculty is to keep admission standards high, because it makes teaching easier; however, this answer excludes some needed groups and will not produce the numbers of nurses that are needed for practice. Education and service must work together in the future to maintain nurse quality and quantity. Nursing education must do more to recruit students and must find innovative methods for teaching a more diverse student body. Nursing service needs to restructure delivery systems in order to use the skills of various types of nurses more effectively, and it needs either to stop doing or, alternatively, to bill for non-nursing services carried out by nurses. Nursing education and nursing practice must work together more closely to define nursing more accurately and to find answers to the pressing problems in both areas.

The NMDS would help meet the challenge to the nurse supply by directly linking education to practice through data generated by patient care. It would formally tie us together through our natural link, the patient. We would work together to set up NISs that would meet multiple needs. Our collective expertise and interaction would make the profession of nursing stronger. Examining and analyzing clinical data through interactive computer systems also provides an alternative teaching method that would assist all types of students. The advantage of computerized information systems and their more advanced cousins, the expert systems, is that they provide some degree of decision support. Manual systems of care planning, even if they use standardized care plans, offer little decision support. Decision aids, such as a pull-up help screen that lists the etiologies and signs and symptoms for a particular diagnosis, are useful for overcoming a short-term memory limitation, help to relate specific information about a particular patient to a general body of knowledge, and facilitate correct decision making. For example, the computer can help a student make a correct nursing diagnosis by comparing patient etiologies, signs, and symptoms, as identified by the student, with the generally accepted etiologies, signs, and symptoms for the average patient with the diagnosis, as identified by nursing experts and stored in the computer.

Faculty

The second major challenge facing nursing education has to do with the fact that very soon all the nursing faculty in universities will be doctorally prepared. These faculty are prepared to do research and advance nursing's knowledge base; in fact, they *must* do this to keep their jobs and to keep nursing a respected discipline. They need time for their research, however; they cannot be both expert clinicians interacting with students 16 to 20 hours a week and expert researchers designing studies, analyzing data, and writing up results. The challenge is to design a new way of teaching undergraduates clinical material that is less expensive but does not compromise quality. The response to this challenge must include a strategy for keeping doctorally prepared faculty in touch with their clinical specialty areas to ensure that their research and teaching remain meaningful.

The NMDS provides part of the answer to this troublesome problem. The use of data sets would make the lengthy and time-consuming teaching-learning care plans we now use obsolete. Through data sets, care planning and student documentation can be monitored in different ways. The use of the computer in clinical teaching also makes possible a new method for teaching decision making, one that perhaps is more effective and less expensive than our current method of role modeling.

The minimum data set would also facilitate the research of both faculty and graduate students. The interaction of faculty with their counterparts in service to develop and refine the data collection systems, to analyze the data, and to test intervention protocols would encourage faculty research, while at the same time promoting quality in the practice setting. The quality assurance programs mandated by the Joint Committee on Accreditation of Hospitals will take on a new step, with clinical problems generated systematically through computer documentation. Those with no known research-based interventions can be referred to faculty colleagues for study (Watson, Bulechek, & McCloskey, 1987).

Curricula

The third challenge has to do with our curricula, which are now in transition. Most schools have abandoned their previous medical models as being too disease- and medicine-dominated; unfortunately, no completely satisfactory replacement has been designed. A survey by De Back (1981) of 270 baccalaureate programs found that none followed a medical model, 19 percent followed a developmental model (organized around concepts of fundamental human needs, as described by the theorists Henderson and Rogers), 6 percent followed an interaction model (organized around the understanding of human interpersonal relationships, as described by the theorists King, Orem, and Orlando), 50 percent followed a systems model (organized around the stability or adaptation of the client, as described by the theorists Johnson, Roy, and Neuman), and 24 percent followed a mixed model (incorporating two or more of the other models). Some of the mixed types, like ours at Iowa, are labeled nursing process curricula.

The use of the nursing process since the 1960s has facilitated the development of nursing knowledge. Professional nursing practice is the diagnosis and treatment of health problems within the scope of nursing. But just what is the scope of nursing? What problems do or should nurses treat? What treatments do or should nurses use? Which treatments work for which diagnoses? Answers to these questions can be more rapidly achieved with the help of a minimum data set implemented through computerized NISs. The main problem will be how to design curricular models that include more nursing content and more help with clinical decision making while still preparing students to function in practice roles that also require physician assistant knowledge and skills.

Part of the solution to this curricular problem is inclusion by faculty of more content on nursing diagnoses, interventions, and outcomes. In the past, the nursing process has been seen mostly as a problem-solving approach—that is, as a process—but implementation of the nursing process with systematic documentation and analysis of the steps also results in products, namely, the diagnoses, interventions, and outcomes that make up nursing content. We need to teach the process of nursing as clinical decision making and the content of nursing as nursing diagnoses and interventions. This immediately leads to several thorny professional questions. What educational preparation is needed to make nursing diagnoses and to carry out and evaluate the interventions? How will the curricula of associate degree programs differ from those of baccalaureate programs? Should faculty be prepared differently for these programs?

With the rapid multiplication of textbooks that use nursing diagnoses, more programs at all levels are including nursing diagnosis content. To my knowledge, however, no one has adopted a nursing diagnosis and intervention curriculum. In such a curriculum, the syllabus would read like a list of nursing diagnoses. For example, the first-year syllabus table of contents would include activity intolerance, alterations in bowel elimination, alterations in comfort, alterations in oral mucous membranes, anxiety, self-care deficit, impairment of skin integrity, sleep pattern disturbance, and so on; these are the diagnoses that are basic to the care of all individuals. The table of contents for the more advanced course in critical care nursing would include ineffective breathing patterns, decreased cardiac output, fluid volume deficit, impaired gas exchange, and so on. A course in health promotion, with clinical experiences in the community, industry, and schools, would include family coping, potential for growth, alteration in heath maintenance, and impaired home maintenance management. A course focused on children as clients would include fear, alterations in family processes, potential for injury, and alterations in parenting. Nursing interventions would be taught as a part of the treatment phase for the nursing diagnoses. Associated medical conditions would be covered, but only as they relate to nursing diagnoses and treatments. Nursing lectures would first cover nursing content—that is, the nursing diagnosis and related treatments—and then discuss related medical conditions.

Perhaps the reason why such a curriculum does not already exist is that nursing diagnoses focus on the independent role of the nurse, whereas in most practice settings nurses also play a collaborative role, in which they carry out the medical treatment plan as prescribed by physicians' orders. The remainder of the solution to the curricular problem lies in continuing to prepare students for these traditional collaborative activities. Many of the skills that we teach in our nursing education program—for example, administration of medications and changing and regulating intravenous fluids—are physician assistant skills which involve implementing the intervention of the physician. Although knowledge and decision-making ability are needed to acquire and use these skills, it is important to recognize that these are not nursing interventions (unless, that is, the nurse has prescribed the medication or the intravenous fluid).

NURSING INTERVENTIONS

In my opinion, it is essential that the NMDS include interventions. A list of nursing interventions defines nursing by detailing what it is that nurses do. This becomes clearer if we think of nursing diagnoses as "belonging" to the patient (since they are patient conditions) and nursing interventions as "belonging" to the nurse (since they are nursing actions). Of course, a list of nursing diagnoses also helps to define nursing, since these are patient conditions, viewed from a nurse's perspective, that can be treated independently by nurses. By itself, however, a list of nursing diagnoses is not a full description of nursing. We need a list or taxonomy of nursing interventions, just as we need one of nursing diagnoses.

There is a great need to identify, label, and classify independent nursing interventions, but any complete list or taxonomy of interventions done by nurses must also include the collaborative activities of the nurse. The NMDS proposes two lists of nursing interventions, which are defined as "actions intended to benefit the patient or client and for which nurses are responsible." Both the definition and the proposed categories include all activities of the nurse. Nursing interventions are included in the preliminary testing of the NMDS, but it has not been decided whether they will be included in the final data set.

The chief obstacle to including interventions in the final NMDS is the lack of a standardized list of interventions. Although we have hundreds of nurse activities in our textbooks, our care plans, and our procedure books, it is still difficult to categorize nursing interventions. Recently, several books (Bulechek & McCloskey, 1985; Synder, 1985) have appeared that make beginning attempts to conceptualize nursing activities. Much work remains to be done in this area, and a number of questions need to be answered. Should a taxonomy of nursing interventions include only the independent interventions? Should assessment activities be included? Should the taxonomy be constructed with a particular theoretical framework in mind? The answers to these questions depend in part on the purpose of the taxonomy. The NMDS provides some direction here, since it was designed for multiple users.

The NMDS will facilitate the identification and categorization of nurse activities. Once we know which interventions nurses perform for which patients, we can study the effectiveness of those interventions. We will be able to determine which patient problems and nursing interventions nurses have the most difficulty with. This information will help us to shape nursing curricula as well as inservice education programs.

CONCLUSION

The key components of the minimum data set are those that focus on nursing care: nursing diagnosis, nursing intervention, nursing outcome, and nursing intensity. Three of the components are steps in the nursing process, which is the framework on which most baccalaureate curricula are based. The collection of standardized data on these steps of the nursing process will help to define nursing as a unique discipline. This benefits nursing education along with the rest of the profession.

REFERENCES

Bulechek, G. M., & McCloskey, J. C. (1985). *Nursing interventions: Treatments for nursing diagnoses.* Philadelphia: W. B. Saunders.

De Back, V. (1981). The relationship between senior nursing students' ability to formulate nursing diagnoses and the curriculum model. *Advances in Nursing Science, 3* (3), 51–66.

Watson, G., Bulechek, G., & McCloskey, J. (1987). *Qumar: Quality assurance model using research.* Unpublished paper, University of Iowa, Iowa City.

Synder, M. (1985). *Independent nursing interventions.* New York: John Wiley & Sons.

Zielstorff, R. D. (1984). Why aren't there more significant automated nursing information systems? *The Journal of Nursing Administration, 14* (1), 7–10.

ACKNOWLEDGMENTS

Elizabeth Swanson and Gloria Bulechek of the University of Iowa offered valuable comments on an earlier draft of this paper.

THE NURSING MINIMUM DATA SET:
BENEFITS AND IMPLICATIONS FOR CLINICAL NURSES

Regina M. Maibusch, MS, RN
Clinical Nurse Specialist
St. Michael's Hospital
Milwaukee, WI

As Werley and Zorn have noted elsewhere in this volume (p. 105), there are 16 elements in the Nursing Minimal Data Set (NMDS) and several levels for structuring these data. At the first level is the narrative record of care, whose format and content are specific to the agency or institution—e.g., problem-oriented recording, focus charting, chronological charting, or flow sheets. Broad standards for information content are set by the general profession, often on the basis of legal experience, the generic standards of the American Nurses' Association, or specialty standards. At the second, or middle-level, is the clinical nursing abstract (CNA), which is standardized by the type of setting in which the nursing is occurring and may be represented by the nursing cover or face sheet (similar to the face sheet currently used in acute care facilities by physicians). The CNA could conceivably be mandated by an accrediting body. Colating information from the CNA could occur, resulting in a third level, regional data. This could be further abstracted to create national data. Through an audit trail, national data could be traced back to the institution or setting where care occurred. Appropriate safeguards of confidentiality need to exist.

Since the aim of this paper is to examine the implications of the NMDS for practitioners, I will address elements 1 through 4 of the NMDS, which collectively are known as the nursing care data. The remaining elements, grouped under the two categories of patient/client demographic data and service data, are more properly the concern of nursing managers and medical records personnel. The four elements of nursing care data that I will consider are nursing diagnoses, nursing interventions, nursing outcomes, and intensity of nursing care.

At this point, it is important to realize that nursing diagnoses, though widely used, are not universally accepted. Nonetheless, problem identification—

the nursing process—has a long history in nursing; in the literature, it first appears in the proceedings of an educational conference held over 35 years ago (McManus, 1951). It will be noted that assessment is not included in the elements of the nursing care data. The Post-Conference Task Force of the NMDS came to a consensus that assessment should be included at the CNA level but not at the NMDS level. Many consider it reasonable to expect nurses to record the assessment data that led to a nursing diagnosis: others hold that the professional nurse should not have to justify a diagnosis within the data set. I believe that a reasonable explanation must be given for any conclusion or nursing diagnosis arrived at, and that there must be a connection between the indicators and the nursing diagnosis. Unless some assessment data are included, the accuracy of a diagnosis cannot be evaluated at a later date.

Nurses must take special pains to be precise and concise when recording patient data; failure to do so would make the data too voluminous and too difficult to abstract. To ask for more data than the census bureau collects, as one expert in the field puts it, would be pointless and wasteful.

Underlying this concept of adequate recording of nursing phenomena is the assumption that appropriate technology will be introduced into more nursing care settings. Computerization of nursing data forces parsimony and precision in expression, as anyone who has ever developed a computer screen knows. Furthermore, because of the sheer volume of the data, information cannot be efficiently retrieved without the appropriate technology. It is essential that we do all the recording of the nursing process, but it is equally essential that the relevant data be stored in an accessible form.

NURSING DIAGNOSES

As pointed out earlier, the first element of the nursing care data is nursing diagnosis, not nursing assessment. The options for the framework of nursing diagnosis content, as agreed on by the Post Conference Task Force, are probably inclusive enough to accommodate all who hold that nursing is the diagnosis and treatment of human responses (American Nurses' Association, 1980). Nurses may subscribe to the North American Nursing Diagnosis Association list or to another diagnostic scheme, such as the Omaha Visiting Nurse Association, Orem, or Carnevali; if none of these are considered adequate, the infinite "other" option can be chosen. This all-inclusiveness bodes well for accommodation of the practice of nurses in all settings—acute care hospital, long-term care facility, joint practice, or independent nurse practice. Whichever option is selected, standardization of procedure is vital. The abstractor must know where to look. Are the nursing diagnoses on a nursing diagnosis or problem list that is an index to the patient record? Or are the nursing diagnoses abstracted from the nursing care plan? Or would the primary nurse be required to list the nursing diagnosis on the CNA (face sheet), as physicians do? (The last is the choice that leads to the most accurate data.)

NURSING INTERVENTIONS

Nursing interventions present a more difficult problem than nursing diagnoses. A system of codification for the intervention nurses practice must be accepted. Two taxonomies of interventions have been proposed through the NMDS Conference, one with 16 elements and the other with seven. The seven-element taxonomy has the following categories: (1) surveillance/observation, (2) supportive measures, (3) assistive measures, (4) treatments/procedures, (5) emotional support, (6) teaching, and (7) coordination of care. Each of these terms has been defined. Inservicing regarding the definitions is imperative, and we must perform repeated reliability testing to maintain accuracy, just as we do for patient classification systems. We argue about which schema of nursing diagnoses we should use—NANDA, Omaha, Orem, Campbell, Carnevali, etc.—because as a profession we have only begun to develop useful taxonomies. Although work has been published such as the Bulechek and McCloskey book on interventions (Bulechek & McCloskey, 1985) we have not collectively grappled with this developmental task. The interventions of physicians are generally grouped under five headings: prescription of medicine, surgery, chemotherapy, radiation, and psychotherapy. We do not yet have such a simple and elegant classification.

It is likely that staff nurses or nurse caregivers in all settings would be willing to categorize their interventions if an adequate taxonomy existed. I am concerned about the numerous interventions that never get recorded, whether because they are a routine, expected part of the nurse-patient interaction, or because they are highly complex, or for some other reason. For example, how does a nurse record the transportation of a patient from a general nursing unit to a critical care unit? Let us apply the seven-element taxonomy mentioned earlier. The activities involved include placing the patient on the cart, moving him or her from one place to another, ongoing surveillance of the vital signs during the move, verbal explanation and support, monitoring the intravenous infusion and all the safety elements involved, seeing that none of the intravenous or endotracheal tubes is accidently removed and that the patient is not physically injured, and perhaps calming the distraught family member, as well as coordinating the care provided by the respiratory therapist, the transport aide, the resident, and several nurses. This single intervention would embrace five of the seven elements: surveillance, supportive measures, assistive measures, emotional support, and coordination of care.

NURSING OUTCOMES

Nursing outcome is defined as the status at discharge of all nursing diagnoses identified during an episode or encounter of care. This could be quite a varied list if many nursing diagnoses had been identified in a patient/client in one hospitalization. The patient might be admitted to the intensive care unit, then transferred to a modified care unit, then moved to a surgical floor, and finally, if complications occurred, returned to the intensive care unit. The NMDS gives several choices for outcome: resolved, unresolved, and referred for further nursing care or a peaceful death. The primary nurse is the best one to make the determination of what occurred, but this poses some problems for the practitioner. In the traditional eight-hour shift, a full-time nurse works five out of twenty-one possible shifts per weeks, which amounts to approximately one fourth of the time that the patient is under the care of nurses in a week. Who is to say what the outcomes are if the patient is discharged unexpectedly? How often must a nurse answer, when asked about a patient, "I don't know, this is the first day I have this patient"?

INTENSITY OF NURSING CARE

Intensity of nursing care involves both nursing staff and management. It is concerned with caregiver mix and hours of patient care time. In an acute care setting with an all-nurse staff on a given shift, there is no caregiver mix, since no practical nurses or nursing assistants are involved in care. In such a situation, a nurse might be assigned six patients. Would each patient be credited for one and a third hours of nurse time on that shift? If, as usually happens, a nurse is assigned to some complex and some less complex patients, how can he or she sort out how much time was given to each patient? Of course, if the nurse carried a computer terminal in her pocket and entered the data as he or she went along, little time would have to be spent determining time allocation at the end of the shift.

CONCLUSION

We need all these data for research. We need national data for clinical studies across settings. Such data collection can be done manually, but it is tedious and very expensive, both in money and in cost of time. Appropriate technology could make it vastly easier to record the data and to retrieve it for research purposes.

All these possibilities are exciting to me as a practitioner. We need testing of the proposed NMDS. We need to inform educators about the concept and motivate them to include it in curricula. We need nursing administrators to see the contribution to nursing research that their institutions can make. We need to generate pride in the direct caregivers, who are now our largest group of nurses. We need to help staff nurses understand that they are the ones who are best able to identify nursing phenomena.

Finally, the NMDS is a challenge to the practitioners of nursing to be precise and concise in recording all the elements of the nursing process: assessment, diagnosis, interventions, outcomes, and, to some extent, intensity of care. The completeness of these data could be greatly enhanced by the implementation of computers for the use of nurses in their day-to-day recording.

REFERENCES

American Nurses' Association. (1980). *Nursing: A social policy statement.* Kansas City, MO: Author.

Bulechek, G. M., & McCloskey, J. C. (1985). *Nursing intervention: Treatments for nursing diagnoses.* Philadelphia: W. B. Saunders.

McManus, R. L. (1951). *Proceedings of nursing education planning conference.* New York: Teacher's College, Columbia University.

PRACTICE

AN UPDATE ON THE NATIONAL COMMISSION ON NURSING IMPLEMENTATION PROJECT: MANAGEMENT OF PRACTICE

Tim Porter-O'Grady, EdD, RN
Senior Health Consultant
Master Consultants, Inc.
Atlanta, GA

It should come as no surprise that the profession of nursing is entering a new era in the delivery of its services in the American health care marketplace. The National Commission on Nursing Implementation Project is now deeply involved in assessing the current status of that marketplace and its needs both as they exist today and as they are likely to exist in the 21st century. The goal of the Project is to be able to identify those characteristics and processes that will exist in the future marketplace and, out of that identification, to develop educational, service, and research strategies that will help the profession of nursing to meet the demands of the time.

The role of the Workgroup on Management of Practice (Workgroup II) is to help to determine, through dialogue, group work, research, case study, and various other methodologies, what the practice setting for the 21st century will be like. It follows that Workgroup II must also attempt to determine where the profession of nursing is today and to pinpoint the activities, strategies, and processes that must be implemented to identify and disseminate those creative models of nursing management and practice in hospitals, health care agencies, and communities that lead to cost-effective, high-quality nursing care (National Commission on Nursing Implementation Projects, 1986).

YEAR 1

The backdrop for much of the deliberations of Workgroup II's first year of work grew out of consideration of the recommendations made by the National Commission on Nursing in 1983. A review of many of the recommendations contained in that report led the workgroup to construct an evaluation model for nursing care delivery in the health care system. That evaluation model served as a framework for developing specific characteristics from which judgments could be made about the appropriateness of the health care delivery system in the context of the 21st century. The characteristics identified by Workgroup II in year 1 relate specifically to cost-effective, high-quality nursing care delivery systems that would meet the future demands of the marketplace. These characteristics center on the health care delivery system, the consumer receiving health care services, the process of delivering those services, and the outcomes associated with the services delivered (in relationship to both the delivery system and the consumer).

YEAR 2

Year 2 of the project focuses on more operational processes that utilize the information and resources developed from the work of year 1. The specific objective for year 2 is to target and develop a plan for influencing the environmental factors that enhance the quality and cost-effectiveness of nursing care delivery systems. With that objective as a starting point, more specific activities have been decided on:

1. Use of a case study method that refines the year 1 characteristics and applies them to the analysis of examples of nursing care delivery systems from across the country;

2. Identification, on the basis of the nursing care delivery system examples, of those factors or specific features that facilitate or inhibit the development or replication of cost-effective, high-quality nursing care systems; and

3. Clear identification and enumeration (in order of priority) of those environmental factors that positively influence or ensure the development and replication of these cost-effective high-quality nursing care delivery systems.

The agenda of Workgroup II for year 2, therefore, has been to bring to fulfillment the work of both year 1 and year 2. It has provided concrete direction to the National Commission on Nursing Implementation Project on specific actions that would move the profession of nursing from its current position in the 20th century to a position where it could proactively address the needs and demands of the health care system in the next century. Workgroup II's membership is necessarily diverse; it includes nurse business persons, educators, researchers, and administrators, as well as individuals from the health care industry at large, representing insurance, health administration, business, and consumers. This diverse representation ensures that the full range of options available to the National Commission on Nursing

Implementation Project will be considered, and that the base of response will be the broadest possible.

Methods

A modified case strategy was selected as an appropriate framework for undertaking site visits and service reporting on various creative and unique approaches to providing health care services, both within and outside the traditional framework of care delivery. Assessment tools have been developed by the workgroup to enable it to evaluate the elements common to these approaches that enhance quality and cost-effectiveness.

Through this process, Workgroup II has reduced the more than 50 essential characteristics of a high-quality cost-effective delivery system that were developed during year 1 to 10 major features that must be consistent within each delivery system. These features include the following:

1. Identifying the role nursing plays in policy formation at the corporate level;
2. The authority over physical and clinical resources for practice;
3. Relationships between and among health providers;
4. The responsiveness of service and system components;
5. The relationship of nursing to payors and the business community;
6. The integration of consumer needs and values;
7. The attraction and retention of appropriately qualified clinical nurse professionals;
8. Appropriate mechanisms for assuring quality and evaluation;
9. The ability to demonstrate cost effectiveness; and
10. The ability of the nursing service to be economically viable within the context in which it is offered.

These features have been further defined by the workgroup, and specific action statements will be generated from them that will guide the nursing leadership. From these action statements are derived specific strategies that are suggested and reported to the nursing and consumer communities, with an eye to achieving the goals identified by NCNIP, specifically in regard to management of practice in the health delivery system. The aim of these strategies is to help create successful models of nursing management and service in hospitals and communities that lead to cost-effective delivery of high-quality nursing care.

Site visits and other reporting mechanisms for evaluating current care models are planned and developed by Workgroup II and assigned to project staff or to workgroup members using the features determined to be essential to any successful model. These sites, therefore, will be further refined.

Those that exemplify major elements of the features will be identified as possible frameworks on which nursing professionals in the field can model organizational and service structures. In this way, the various models that have proved successful or have demonstrated appropriate transitional value and that can motivate nurses to confront the future can then be utilized or adapted in a wider range of settings across the country. Such replication helps to ensure the utilization of successful and appropriate models for rendering high-quality service and cost-effective delivery of health care.

Resulting Strategies

The efforts of Workgroup II have also resulted in a variety of other strategies that, when addressed and incorporated into the process of developing appropriate health care services for the future, have unique value. The strategies cover a wide range of applicable issues: the appropriate distribution of technical and professional programs offered in nursing, case management systems, professional nursing management of care, marketplace responses to a changing health care delivery system, work environments that are structured to support professional nursing practice, use of public forums to describe economic and service viability and the need for response to the consumer population, the development of the role of the nursing administrator, the response of the institution, the organization of the system to meet the needs of nursing, and the importance of making nursing a more viable career. These and other strategies have been incorporated within a broader picture that requires nursing to assume a wide variety of responsibilities in the delivery system in ways not currently available or in creative structures that have yet to be conceived. They will be addressed in detail in the report of the Second Invitational Conference of the National Commission on Nursing Implementation Project.

CONCLUSIONS

Clearly, the work of the National Commission on Nursing Implementation Project, and specifically the work of Workgroup II, has been challenging, demanding, and creative. The energies of the best minds in nursing and health care have been brought together for serious deliberation on the state of the health care delivery system, the changes leading us into newer frameworks for the delivery of services, the economic realities of change, and, ultimately, the construction of the vision of the health care delivery system of the 21st century. The workgroup has identified the strategies that can enable nursing to cope wth the realities of the new delivery system and to have in place appropriately prepared practitioners who can confront the realities of a changing marketplace and take a leading role in deciding how it will unfold and how services will be provided. The true satisfaction in this project is to watch the deliberations of a wide variety of professionals in nursing and in many other fields as they consider how best to proactively address the issues confronting the health care marketplace.

It is anticipated that in year 3 of the project the NCN will make use of the implementation strategies, processes, models, and suggestions formulated and move from deliberation into action. The NCNIP will begin to undertake the strategies that will ensure implementation of processes which move nursing to respond to the health care needs identified. It becomes clear that nursing is dealing with the realities of change in a mature and studied manner. Through the work of the NCNIP a blueprint has been developed that ensures that the profession of nursing, through its forums, institutions, and services, will respond to the needs of the future in a consolidated and meaningful manner.

REFERENCES

National Commission on Nursing. (1983). *Summary report and recommendations.* Chicago, IL: Author.

National Commission on Nursing Implementation Project. (1986). *Invitational conference report.* Milwaukee, WI: Author, pp. 27–46.

TYPICAL PATTERNS OF NURSING PRACTICE

Marjory Peterson, EdD, RN
Assistant Professor
School of Nursing
Rutgers University
Newark, NJ

Nurses claim that one of their major contributions to the health care system and its clients is caring and genuine concern, which function as antidotes to a depersonalized, dehumanized system (Maraldo, 1982). Ideal nursing practice is described as flexible, compassionate, skilled, and based on scientific knowledge. Typical nursing practice, however, has been described as technical, inflexible and unengaged, characterized by nurses' avoidance of most patients (Flaskerud, Halloran, Janken, Lund, & Zetterland, 1979; Davitz & Davitz, 1981; Benner, 1984; Peterson, 1987; Joel, 1982-1987).

Research into nurse-patient relationships and selected variables that may affect these relationships has been extensive. The findings of such studies, unfortunately, have little conceptual or operational relationship to one another. Nurses' personal traits, education, experience, and knowledge have not been conclusively shown to influence the quality of nursing practice (Allen, 1981; Benner, 1984; Cohen, 1980; Davitz & Davitz, 1981; Pearlmutter, 1973); however, in two separate small studies of especially empathetic nurses, the factor common to all study nurses was the high personal satisfaction nurses gained from nursing practice, which they viewed as a professional worthwhile career (Benner, 1984; Davitz & Davitz, 1981).

The most salient factor to emerge from a vast literature on the quality of nurse-patient relationships is that the value nurses place on clinical nursing may be an important influence on their nursing practice.

STUDY RATIONALE AND METHODS

Groups and social theorists consider that members of workgroups adapt their personal value systems to fit in with the norms and values of their workgroup (Cartwright & Zander, 1960; Parsons, 1956; Radcliffe-Brown,

1952; Shaw, 1976). The norms and values of a group are expressed in the typical acceptable modes of behavior that members use in interaction with each other and in obtaining desired workgroup outcomes.

Several studies have noted that nurses are very sensitive to workgroup norms and values and tend to adapt their personal norms and values to those of the clinical workgroup to which they belong (Kramer, 1974, 1981; Peterson, 1983; Peterson, 1987; Stull, 1986). Nurses have been demonstrated to have a sense of accomplishment when acting in conformity with workgroup norms (Peterson, 1983); moreover, as members of a predominately female profession, they may have a tendency to seek consensus and avoid conflict (Gilligan, 1982). Nurses select their workgroup norms and values from diverse and contradictory messages sent by the lay public, the medical community, nursing administrators, and nurse educators (Christman, 1979; Kramer, 1981; Muff, 1982). Clinical nurses do not seem to have arrived at a consensus on their proper role and function (Evans, Fitzpatrick, & Howard-Rubern, 1983; McClure, 1984).

Group leaders play a major role in the selection and enforcement of a group's norms and values (Cartwright & Zander, 1960; Horowitz, 1970; Radcliffe-Brown, 1952). Head nurses, who are the group leaders of most small groups of practicing clinical nurses, have been noted to exert considerable influence on the values and the practice norms of the nurses whom they supervise (Bergman, Stockler, Shavit, Sharon, Feinberg, & Damon, 1981; Duxbury, Armstrong, Drew, & Henley, 1984; Joel, 1982–87; Johnston, 1983; Peterson, 1987).

These constructs from group dynamics were used as the theoretical rationale in the design of a study that would examine nursing practice from the perspective of group dynamics. In this study, I examined the norms and values of three groups of nurses. Each group of nurses was observed for five to six weeks while working on one of three selected medical floors in the same hospital. All three units utilized a system of primary nursing, and their patient populations and staffing patterns were similar. The external similarities of the floors allowed for attribution of differences in nursing practice to internal group dynamics on each floor rather than to external variables.

The norms and values related to typical nursing practice were inferred from observation and analysis of the nurses' interactions with each other, with patients, and with other hospital personnel. This method of research has been named grounded theory (Glaser & Strauss, 1967; Stern, 1980). In this approach, the researcher works within a matrix instead of following a series of linear steps. An ongoing comparison was made between each interaction and each other interaction and between the typical pattern of interaction on each unit with the typical patterns of interaction on the other two units. This technique of constant comparison made it possible to identify typical behavior patterns, as well as nurses' explicit and implicit expectations, orientations, beliefs, and attitudes. Differences and similarities between the three groups were explained in terms of group dynamics.

FINDINGS

Norms and Values Common to All Study Nurses

Group Influences on Nursing Practice. Each group of nurses' psychosocial nursing practice was influenced by group norms and values. On all three units, the nurses functioned as a group, with more than two thirds behaving in a typical fashion that reflected the group's shared norms and values. Nurses who were atypical in their behavior and attitudes were recognized as deviant by their group and were penalized for this deviance in various subtle ways (e.g., a heavier workload or fewer primary patients). The deviant nurses on each unit fell evenly into two categories: nurses who were more empathetic than the typical nurses and nurses who were less empathetic than the typical nurses.

Influence of Group Leader. In two of the three groups, the head nurse was the group leader and had a major influence on the selection and enforcement of the group's norms and values. The third group did not accept the head nurse or anyone else as a leader. This group had failed to achieve work-oriented goals.

The nurses' morning routine and the typical approach to patients on two of the units were clearly influenced by the norms of the head nurse. On unit 1, the head nurse's insistence that all morning care be finished on time created a rushed, tense atomosphere. On unit 2, the head nurse's insistence that medical orders be given top priority in patient care led to the nurses regarding this as their priority and reminding each other to check and implement medical orders frequently. On units 1 and 2, the nurses emulated the head nurse's style of uniform. On unit 3, the nurses flagrantly violated the very flexible dress code set by the head nurse.

The staff nurses in all three groups had difficulty in establishing collaborative relationships with other health professionals; in each group, the head nurse carried out this function for the group. The head nurses on all three units usually attended some part of medical rounds, but the staff nurses rarely did, even when they had time and their primary patients were involved in the discussion.

Typical Behavior Patterns. On all three units, typical care was usually limited to physical care, technical procedures, and the administration of medications. Each group of nurses had developed a morning routine/protocol that facilitated the typical approach to patients. Only patients who required extensive physical nursing care or specialized care had the opportunity for frequent interactions with nurses.

A typical interaction with a patient who required extensive nursing care was as follows:

> NURSE: I have come to wash you.
> PATIENT: Okay.
> NURSE: Did your son visit last night?
> PATIENT: Yes, but he didn't stay long...
> NURSE: Mm.
> *(The remainder of patient care was given in silence, except for brief instructions to the patient from nurse and some conversation between the nurse and a nursing aide who came into the room to ask a question.)*

Patients admitted for extensive diagnostic procedures often became extremely anxious and sought out nurses, but they were rarely approached by a nurse. The following is an example of a typical interaction with a patient admitted for diagnostic tests:

> *(The patient, a 44-year-old woman who had undergone a bronchoscopy the previous day, paced her room, then sat on her bed; she was in tears.)*
> PATIENT *(to other patients in room):* I can't go, it's too much after yesterday. *(Nurses entered and left the four-bed room without comment.)* *(The patient saw the dietitian at the nursing station and rushed up to her.)*
> PATIENT: Why do I have a liquid diet again? I can't go for another test today. *(The patient started to cry again.)*
> *(The dietitian looked in the patient's chart.)*
> DIETITIAN: Its a CAT scan today; that doesn't hurt. You just lie there. *(The patient returned to bed.)*
> PATIENT: *(to a nurse in the room):* I get so upset, you must think I'm always making a fuss.
> *(The nurse smiled and said nothing.)*

Typical nurses, more empathetic nurses, and less empathetic nurses interacted with patients in markedly different ways.

> The patient was an elderly woman who was a little confused at times but could carry on a rational conversation. She required a daily dressing for a foot ulcer.
> *1. Empathetic nurse:*
> NURSE: I have come to dress your foot.
> PATIENT: Can you cut the tape [on the old dressing]?

NURSE: Okay, sweetie, I'll be gentle. *(The nurse smiled at patient and redressed patient's foot, maintaining eye contact all the while.)*
PATIENT: It's not so painful today as usual.
NURSE: There now, sweetie, it's all done. *(The nurse smiled at patient and left room.)*
2. *Typical nurse:*
NURSE: It's time for your dressing now.
PATIENT: She usually does it later.
NURSE: Well, she's not here today, I'm in charge. *(The nurse dressed the patient's foot while standing at the patient's side, thus making eye contact difficult, then left room without further comment. She did not seem to notice the patient's grimaces of pain during the dressing.)*
3. *Less empathetic nurse:*
(The nurse entered the patient's room and did not speak at all to the patient while dressing her foot.)
PATIENT *(in tears):* Ow, ow, that hurts.
(The nurse kept her back to the patient during the dressing and showed no response to patient's cries of pain and tears.)

On all three units, patients' requests for physical nursing assistance or for symptomatic relief were met reasonably, appropriately and promptly, if these requests were made in a coherent and polite manner. On all three units, patients' incoherent expressions of distress were usually ignored. Patients who exhibited disruptive behavior were referred to other health professionals (e.g., social workers) without delay.

An example of a typical incident involving patients' requests will illustrate typical nurse responses. A patient admitted for cardiac catheterization requested internal sanitary tampons prior to preparation for this invasive diagnostic test. No tampons were available, and the patient became upset, wept, and screamed. When one of the nurses gave the patient a tampon from her personal supply, the patient became calmer and went for the test as scheduled. The nurses mentioned at social work rounds that the patient was a "case" for the social worker, since she seemed to "get hysterical" at times.

Orientations, Beliefs, Attitudes, and Expectations

On all three units nurses were expected to demonstrate an understanding of physiologic and psychosocial theory, either in formal or informal discussions about patients or in written care plans. There was, however, no observable expectation that nurses would apply this theoretical knowledge to their daily nursing practice. For example, on one unit the nurses were knowledgable about the acquired immune deficiency syndrome (AIDS) and had developed a model care plan for patients with this disease that addressed physiologic and psychosocial aspects of nursing care. Nevertheless, one nurse expressed astonishment when told at a staff meeting that a young woman whom she had been looking after for four days had AIDS (as an admission diagnosis). On another unit, nurses discussed in detail the psychopathology of a young male patient, linking it to his troubled home life and the recent death of his father. Nevertheless, the nurses continued to avoid interaction with the patient and to rely on the crisis team and inappropriate coercion to deal with his disruptive behavior.

On all three units nurses used social/moral assessment of patients. A significant part of this social/moral valuing was nurses' telling each other anecdotes concerning patients. These anecdotes facilitated one group's humane and two groups' dehumanizing nurse-patient interactions.

In group meetings on all three units, nurses discussed scheduling, medical practice, pathophysiology, psychopathology, and abstract nursing issues (such as model nursing care plans). Rarely, however, did they discuss actual daily nursing practice.

Norms and Values: Unit 1

Unit 1 nurses were characterized by efficiency, neatness, and politeness. These nurses' typical approach to patients was cool, polite, and neutral. Patients were given physical care that ranged from adquate to excellent. The unit 1 protocols resulted in the nurses' being rushed and spending only one to two hours in the patients' rooms each morning. Unit 1 nurses focused on task-oriented rather than person-oriented nursing. Nurses were expected to be calm and polite to patients at all times.

Typical Behavior Patterns. A typical nurse–patient interaction on unit 1 might proceed as follows:

> *(A patient was angry and shouted at nurses at the nurses' desk because a transporter was waiting to take her for a test and she had not had a necessary injection.)*
> PATIENT: I will have to be here an extra day: it's not fair.
> NURSE: I will get the shot now, and the transporter will return later.
> PATIENT: Will he? I can't stay an extra day.
> *(The nurse did not respond but prepared the injection and gave it to the tearful, angry patient without further comment.)*

The following is a typical situation.

> A blind, febrile, middle-aged woman had been admitted during the night. In the morning she repeatedly rang her call bell for a nurse. The nurse told her twice to wait and on the third occasion disconnected the bell. The nurse gave the patient adequate care when her "turn" came.

Orientations, Beliefs, Attitudes, and Expectations: Unit 1

Nurses expected each other to give patients a high standard of physical care and to document and report patients' physical status in detail. There was consternation when it was found that a new nurse had gone off duty without recording her (stable) patient's blood pressure. No similar expectation about documenting patients' emotional status existed.

The unit 1 nurses told each other anecdotes which subtly devalued a patient's social worth if the patient was "difficult" or noncompliant. The following are typical.

> The nurses were sitting in the coffee room. A nurse mimicked an elderly woman who had requested to be put back to bed, saying "If you girls knew how my back hurts you wouldn't make me sit in this chair so long." The other nurses laughed.
>
> A nurse came into the coffee room and remarked about assigned patients, three of whom were terminally ill, "They are all awful in that room; I can't bear to go in there at all. I just put my head in, that's enough." The other nurses nodded sympathetically.

Unit 1 nurses accepted the head nurse as their leader and tried hard to meet her exacting standards for physical patient care and her norm of "finishing" care on time. Empathetic nurses were teased about being "soft" with patients and given a heavy workload on this unit. Less empathetic nurses were given less primary patients than was usual (a subtle insult).

Norms and Values: Unit 2

Unit 2 nurses were characterized by friendly attitudes, peer support, and a rather casual attitude to clothes and nursing techniques. These nurses typically approached patients in a friendly, superficial manner. Patients were usually given adequate physical nursing care. The unit 2 protocols resulted in patients being cared for in a leisurely manner, with nurses spending three hours or more in the patients' rooms each morning. Unit 2 nurses focused on the enactment of medical orders and person-oriented nursing.

Typical Behavior Patterns.   A typical nurse–patient interaction on unit 2 might proceed as follows.

> *(A middle-aged woman with a terminal illness was seated beside her bed.)*
> PATIENT: I feel weak. I think I'm going to throw up.
> NURSE *(smiling):* After all the care we took to make you pretty! We even put a flower in your hair.
> PATIENT *(smiling weakly):* Can I go back to bed?
> NURSE: Sure, that's okay.

The following is a typical situation.

> A nurse had given morning care to one patient, which included changing the patient's colostomy bag. The nurse was now bathing another patient in the four-bed room. The colostomy patient called out, "My bag has burst, it's a mess." The nurse smiled, sighed, and left the second patient in the middle of the bath to get a tray of equipment. She then proceeded to reapply the colostomy bag. The nurse said, "It's my fault; I just can't get the hang of it." After reapplying the colostomy device, the nurse went for morning coffee, returning 20 minutes later to the second patient, who was in disarray awaiting the completion of his morning toilet.

Orientations, Beliefs, Attitudes, and Expectations: Unit 2

The nurses expected each other to give patients an adequate standard of physical nursing care. They expected that this care would be adequately documented. Each patient was expected to have a written nursing care plan. Strict enactment and documentation of medical orders and preparation for medical procedures was expected of all nurses. The head nurse regularly checked that any medical orders, especially preparation for procedures, had been carried out as specified. The nurses reminded each other and cross-checked to make sure that medical orders and care plans had been completed as required.

Nurses were expected to be friendly and cheerful to patients at all times, even when this was inappropriate (e.g., with patients who were tearful and distressed). Nurses were expected to tell anecdotes about patients and their interactions with patients that showed the nurse to be human and warm. The following is typical.

> A nurse, sitting in the coffee room, told other nurses about a blind patient who had died unexpectedly. She said, "He asked me to do everything, wouldn't even wash his face. I said, 'Are your hands disabled?' He said, 'No, but my eyes are.' He was real mean. So I just did everything for him....He was okay when we went off duty."

Empathetic nurses on this unit were respected and, though often assigned sicker patients, were allowed more autonomy in practice and fewer patients in their daily assignment. Less empathetic nurses were often assigned patients in rooms at the end of the unit and sometimes had difficulty getting assistance and support from the other nurses for such things as transfers of helpless, heavy patients. The head nurse was regarded by the nurses as their leader, and she carefully supervised the nurses' practice, particularly with respect to the enactment of medical orders and the nurses' attitudes towards patients.

Norms and Values: Unit 3

Unit 3 nurses were characterized by quarrelsomness, fashionable clothes, and the predominance of student-like attitudes and social rather than work-related behaviors. These nurses' typical approach to patients was a brusque, impersonal one. Patients usually received adequate physical care, but this was rendered by nursing aides and not by the nurses themselves. The protocols on unit 3 limited the contact the nurses had with most patients to specialized procedures and medications. The unit 3 nurses expected that the aides would give most of the physical nursing care except when patients were critically ill or had very specialized technical needs (e.g., when patients were on respirators).

Typical Patterns of Behavior. A typical nurse–patient interaction on unit 3 might proceed as follows.

> *(An elderly Jewish rabbi with a gangrenous ulcer on his foot had just had his hair and beard trimmed by the barber.)*
> PATIENT: Now you can see how I looked when I was young, nurse.
> NURSE: I wouldn't have been interested. I wasn't born then.

The following is a typical situation.

> A patient was admitted during the night because of fluid in her lung. In the morning, a nurse was assigned to give morning care, but she asked an aide to look after the patient. The aide gave the patient morning care. Later that day, the nurses expressed dismay and astonishment when asked about the patient's chest tube drain: "She has a dressing? On her chest?"

Orientations, Beliefs, Attitudes and Expectations: Unit 3

Nurses expected each other to have a detailed knowledge of patients' pathophysiology and psychosocial concerns and to document this in each patient's chart. They did not seem able to apply this knowledge to their daily nursing practice.

The nurses' anecdotes about patients reflected social and moral disapproval of patients who tried to establish social relationships with the nurses or who challenged the nurses' authority in any way. The following is typical.

> The nurses at the nursing desk were discussing a patient, a nun, who was concerned about her discharge plans. One nurse said, "Who would have thought a nun would carry on like that? I guess they get up to all sorts in convents these days." The listening nurses giggled.

On this unit, empathetic nurses received a very heavy work load, in both quantity and quality, often including patients who were on respirators or who required other specialized care. Less empathetic nurses were often assigned duties that relieved them from direct patient care (e.g., library release time to research care plans). Unit 3 nurses did not accept the head nurse as a leader, but they did expect her to help them with physical patient care when this was complex.

Summary

On the whole, the nurses studied were very sensitive to work group norms and values and susceptible to leadership values. They were knowledgeable about psychosocial care but their practice was based primarily on assessment of and meeting patients' needs for physical nursing care. They tended to assess patients socially as acceptable or nonacceptable before deciding to have ordinary friendly or accepting relationships with them. Patients found wanting were dehumanized through anecdotes and treated as "other" by the nurses.

DISCUSSION

Nurses' Sensitivity to Workgroup Norms and Values

The findings suggest that nurses are sensitive to work group norms and values and utilize indirect ways of dealing with deviants. It could be speculated that the nurses' avoidance of direct discussion about their practice and of direct confrontation of deviants was related to the finding that women tend to seek consensus and avoid conflict in their social and work relationships (Gilligan, 1982).

A more immediate cause for nurses' reluctance to confront work related problems, however, may be the difficulties involved in dealing with a system of nursing care delivery that has unrealistic expectations. Despite the existence of primary nursing on all three units, the nurses looked to the head nurse to coordinate nursing and other health care for patients. Although 24-hour responsibility for each patient was assigned to one nurse, in reality nurses had little control over patients' 24-hour care. Patients and other health professionals tended to perceive (correctly, in this particular setting) that nursing care was the responsibility of the group of nurses rather than of one designated nurse. The time dilemma in the institutional setting, where the patient is present for 168 hours a week but the nurse for only 35, has seemingly not been resolved by nursing theorists or by primary nursing care delivery systems.

Nurses' Role Perception and Enactment

The nurses' tendency to limit their functions to physical care, technical procedures, and the giving of medicines suggested that they had a very narrow view of the scope of nursing practice. Two of the groups of nurses in this study did not seem to perceive caring for a sick person's bodily functions as part of nursing but either focused on it entirely (unit 1) or rejected it (unit 3). Despite an emphasis by nursing leaders on integrating psychosocial and physical care in a unique way, these nurses focused predominantly on the area of physical care. These findings may reflect the nursing profession's long struggle with paradoxical perceptions of caring for another's body as being at the same time demeaning and an awesome privilege (Diers, 1984; Nightingale, 1859/1957).

It was observed that although patients admitted for diagnostic procedures became increasingly anxious, they did not seek assistance from nurses. Patients who required extensive physical nursing care became less anxious, despite a paucity of overt psychosocial care. These observations could be accounted for by assuming that the patients did not expect anything more than physical care from nurses. The physical care given by nurses, along with their "thereness" (Stevens, 1979; Winnicott, 1964), may have met some of the patients' expectations of nurses. This idea was negatively supported by the comments of a patient on unit 3. He complained of feeling trapped and alone in a place where "no one cares." The unit 3 nurses were not "there" for patients in this way; they did not render physical care to patients but delegated it to aides.

Social Assessment and Psychosocial Nursing Care

The finding that coherent requests for assistance or symptomatic medication were met but incoherent requests or nonverbal distress were not answered confutes earlier findings suggesting that nurses judge and validate patient's suffering before intervention (McCaffery, 1979). The nurses in this study did judge patients, but they used a social, not a physical, perspective. This finding was reinforced by the social/moral tone of the anecdotes told on each unit, which mirrored each group of nurses' attitudes towards patients. Anecdotes as a way of conferring social value on patients, which then translates into levels of psychosocial care and nurses' involvement with patients, has been previously documented by Glaser and Strauss (1964) in a study of nurses and terminally ill patients.

Nurses on two units utilized anecdotes as a way of "dehumanizing" patients, thus justifying the nurses' avoidance of the patient. Nurses on one unit tried to meet patients' psychosocial needs in a rather superficial manner. These phenomena may reflect the dehumanizing effect of a large institution on both nurse and patient, as well as the nurses' difficulties with the delivery of psychosocial care (Howard, 1975).

The findings seem to support previous research suggesting that there is a great need for the development of a body of supportive practical nursing skills that can be utilized with patients in distress (Davitz & Davitz, 1981; Gardner, 1979; Schoenhofer, 1984). Nurses need guidance on how to provide compassionate humane care while maintaining the personhood of both nurse and patient within the complex modern health care facility.

CONCLUSIONS

Four conclusions can be reached on the basis of this study.

1. There is a need for a model of nursing practice in the institutional setting that encompasses group dynamics and nurses' susceptibility to group norms and values and group leadership. The model would acknowledge the concept that patients in institutions are usually cared for by nurses rather than a nurse. This model should address the discrepancy between the 168-hour week of the patient and the 35-hour work week of the nurse (Peterson, 1987).

2. There is an urgent need for the development of practical supportive nursing interventions for distressed patients that can be easily taught and utilized in complex clinical settings.

3. Further research on the use and effect of patient anecdotes in nursing is needed.

4. A teaching-nursing protocol for nurses to utilize with patients scheduled for invasive diagnostic tests might serve the same purpose that preoperative protocols currently serve, namely, reducing patient anxiety.

REFERENCES

Allen, S. A. K. (1981). An anthropological study of nurse-patient interactions. *Dissertation Abstracts International, 42* (2), 563B. (University Microfilms No. 81-16152).

Altschul, A. T. (1972). *Patient-nurse interaction: A study of interaction patterns in acute psychiatric wards.* London: Churchill & Livingston.

American Nurses' Association. Commission on Nursing Services. (1978). *Roles, responsibilities and qualifications for nursing administrators,* New York: ANA.

Benner, P. (1984). *From novice to expert: Excellence and power in clinical nursing practice.* Reading, MA: Addison-Wesley pp. 402-407.

Bergman, R., Stockler, R. A., Shavit, N., Sharon, N., Feinberg, D., & Danon, A. (1981). Role, selection and preparation of unit head nurses: I, II, & III. *International Journal of Nursing Studies, 18* (2), 123-152; *18* (3), 191-211; *18* (4), 237-250.

Blaylock, J. N. (1970). Characteristics of nurses and of medical-surgical patients to whom they react positively and negatively. *Dissertation Abstracts International, 31* (8), 4796B. (University Microfilms No. 71–05569).

Bogdan, R., & Taylor, S. J. (1975). *Introduction to qualitative research methods: A phenomenological approach to the social sciences.* New York: Wiley.

Cartwright, D., & Zander, A. (1960). Leadership and group performance: Introduction. In D. Cartwright & A. Zander (Eds.). *Group dynamics: Research and theory* (2nd ed.). Evanston, IL: Harper & Row.

Chin, R. (1969). The utility of systems models and developmental models for practitioners. In W. G. Bennis, K. D. Benne, & R. Chin (Eds.). *The planning of change: Readings in the applied behavioral sciences* (2nd ed.). New York: Holt, Rinehart and Winston.

Christman, L. (1979). Professional nursing practice: Impediments to practice. *The Journal of the New York State Nurses' Association, 10* (4), 25–29.

Cohen, B. J. (1980). The perception of patient adaptation to haemodialysis: A study of registered nurses and haemodialysis patients. *Dissertation Abstracts International, 41* (1), 129B. (University Microfilms No. 80–15068).

Copp, L. A. (1974, March). The spectrum of suffering. *American Journal of Nursing,* pp. 491–495.

Davitz, J. R., & Davitz, L. L. (1981). *Inferences of patients' pain and psychological suffering: Studies of nursing behaviors.* New York: Springer.

Diers, D. (1984). To profess: To be a professional. *The Journal of The New York State Nurses' Association, 15* (4), 22–29.

Duxbury, M. L., Armstrong, G. D., Drew, D. J., & Henley, S. J. (1984). Head nurse leadership style with staff nurse burnout and job satisfaction in neonatal intensive care units. *Nursing Research, 33* (2), 97–101.

Evans, D., Fitzpatrick, T., Howard-Rubern, J. (1983). A district takes action. *American Journal of Nursing, 83* (1), 52–54.

Fagerhaugh, S. Y., & Strauss, A. (1977). *Politics of pain management: Staff-patient interaction.* Menlo Park, CA: Addison-Wesley.

Flaskerud, J. H., Halloran, E. J., Janken, J., Lund, M., & Zetterland, J. (1979). Avoidance and distancing: A descriptive view of nursing. *Nursing Forum, 18* (2), 158–174.

Gardner, K. G. (1979). Supportive nursing: A critical review of the literature. *Psychiatric Nursing, 17* (10), 10–16.

Gilligan, C. (1982). *In a different voice: Psychological theory and women's development.* Cambridge, MA: Harvard University Press.

Glaser, B. G. (1978). *Theoretical sensitivity: Advances in the methodology of grounded theory.* Available from author, P.O. Box 143, Mill Valley, CA 94941.

Glaser, B. G., & Strauss, A. L. (1964, June). The social loss of dying patients. *American Journal of Nursing,* pp. 119–121.

Glaser, B. G., & Strauss, A. L. (1967). *The discovery of grounded theory: Strategies for qualitative research.* New York: Aldine.

Hammond, K. R. (1966). Clinical inference in nursing. *Nursing Research, 15,* 236–243.

Hall, L. (1966). Another view of nursing care and quality. In K. M. Straub & K. S. Parker (Eds.), *Continuity of patient care: The role of nursing.* Washington, DC: Catholic University Press.

Hargreaves, W. A., & Runyon, N. (1969). Patterns of psychiatric nursing: Role differences in nurse–patient interaction. *Nursing Research, 18* (4), 300–307.

Hinshaw, A. S., & Atwood, J. R. (1982). A patient satisfaction instrument: Precision by replication. *Nursing Research, 31* (3), 170–175.

Horowitz, J. J. (1970). *Team practice and the specialist: An introduction to interdisciplinary teamwork.* Springfield, IL: Thomas.

Howard, J. (1975). Humanization and dehumanization of health care: A conceptual view. In J. Howard & A. Strauss (Eds.), *Humanizing health care.* New York: Wiley.

Joel, L. (1987). Rutgers College of Nursing. Teaching nursing home projects annual reports, 1982–87. Available from the Robert Wood Johnson Foundation. New Brunswick, New Jersey.

Johnston, P. F. (1983, November). Head nurses as middle managers. *The Journal of Nursing Administration, 16,* 22–26.

Kramer, M. (1974). *Reality shock: Why nurses leave nursing.* St. Louis: C. V. Mosby.

Kramer, M. (1981). Why does reality shock continue? In G. C. McClosky & H. K. Grace (Eds.), *Current issues in nursing practice.* Boston, MA: Blackwell Scientific.

La Monica, E. L. (1979). *The Nursing process: A humanistic approach,* Menlo Park, CA: Addison–Wesley.

Lorber, J. (1975). Good patients and problem patients: Conformity and deviance in a general hospital. *Journal of Health and Social Behavior, 16* (2), 213–225.

McCaffery, M. (1979). *Nursing management of the patient with pain* (2nd ed.). Philadelphia: J. B. Lippincott.

McClure, M. (1984, March). Managing the professional nurse: II. Applying management theory to the challenges. *The Journal of Nursing Administration,* pp. 11–17.

Maraldo, P. (1982). Nurse on your mark, get set, go, *The Calendar of The New York State Nurses' Association, 42* (2), 4.

Merton, R. K. (1964). *Social theory and social structure.* London: The Free Press of Glencoe.

Moores, B., & Grant, G. B. W. (1976). On the nature and incidence of staff–patient interactions in hospitals for the mentally handicapped. *International Journal of Nursing Studies, 13,* 69–81.

Muff, J. (1982). Handmaiden, battle-axe, whore: An exploration into the fantasies, myths and stereotypes about nurses. In J. W. Muff (Ed.), *Socialization, sexism, and stereotyping: Women's issues in nursing.* St. Louis, C. V. Mosby.

Nightingale, F. (1957/1859). *Notes on nursing: What it is, and what it is not.* Philadelphia: J. B. Lippincott.

Oberst, M. T. (1982). Research and clinical realities: A commentary on evaluative study of primary nursing. *The Journal of The New York State Nurses' Association, 13* (2), 23–25.

Oiler, C. (1982). The phenomenological approach in nursing research, *Nursing Research, 31,* 178–181.

Parsons, T. (1956). Suggestions for a sociological approach to the theory of organizations. *Administrative Science Quarterly, 1,* 63–69, 74–80.

Paton, X., & Stirling, E. (1974). Frequency and type of dyadic nurse–patient verbal interactions in a mental subnormality hospital. *International Journal of Nursing Studies, 11,* 135–145.

Pearlmutter, D. R. (1973). Towards a definition of emotional support. *Dissertation Abstracts International, 34* (5), 2279A. (University Microfilms No. 73-25167).

Peterson, M. (1987, May). Time and the nursing process. *Holistic Nursing Practice, 1* (3), 72–80.

Peterson, M. F. (1983). Co-workers and hospital staffs' work attitudes: Individual difference moderators. *Nursing Research, 32* (2), 115–120.

Peterson, M. (1985). The norms and values held by three groups of nurses concerning psycho-social nursing practice. Unpublished doctoral dissertation, Teachers College, Columbia University, New York.

Pinneo, R. (1982). Evaluative study of primary nursing. *The Journal of New York State Nurses' Association, 13* (2), 20–22.

Radcliffe-Brown, A. E. (1952). *Structure and function in primitive society.* London: Oxford University Press.

Rickleman, B. L. (1971). Characteristics of nurses and of psychiatric patients to whom they react positively and negatively. *Dissertation Abstracts International, 32* (2), 841A. (University Microfilms No. 71-20026).

Ritvo, M. M. (1963). Who are good and bad patients? *Modern Hospital, 100,* 79-81.

Schatzman, L., & Strauss, L. A. (1973). *Field research: Strategies for a natural sociology.* Englewood, NJ: Prentice-Hall.

Schoenhofer, S. (1984). Support as a legitimate nursing action. *Nursing Outlook, 32* (4), 218-219.

Shaw, M. E. (1976). *Group dynamics: The psychology of small group behavior* (2nd ed.). New York: McGraw-Hill.

Stern, N. P. (1980). Grounded theory methodology: Its uses and processes. *Image, 12* (1), 20-23.

Stevens, B. J. (1979). *Nursing theory: Analysis, application, evaluation.* Boston: Little, Brown & Co.

Stockwell, F. (1972). The unpopular patient. *Monographs of the Royal College of Nursing* (No. 2, Series 1).

Stull, M. P. (1986). Staff nurse performance: Effects of goal setting and performance feedback. *Journal of Nursing Administration, 16* (7), 26-30.

Summers, . (1979, September). Give your patient more personal space. *Nursing '79,* p. 56.

Van Maanen, J. (1979a). Reclaiming qualitative methods for organizational research: A preface. *Administrative Science Quarterly, 24* (4), 527-538.

Van Maanen, J. (1979b). The fact of fiction in social ethnography. *Administrative Science Quarterly, 24* (4), 539-550.

White, M. (1972). Importance of selected nursing activities. *Nursing Research, 21* (1), 4-14.

Wilson-Barnett, J. (1976). Stress in hospital: Patients' psychological reaction to illness and health care. *Journal of Advanced Nursing, 1,* 351-358.

Winnicott, D. W. (1964). *The child, the family and the outside world.* London: Penguin.

Wolcott, H. (1975). Criteria for an ethnographic approach to research in schools. *Human Organizations, 34,* 111-127.

THE NURSING PRESENCE EXAMINED BY ASSESSING JOINT PRACTICE

Hans O. Mauksch, PhD
Professor Emeritus, University of Missouri/Columbia
Lecturer, Sociology, University of Georgia, Athens

James D. Campbell, PhD,
Assistant Professor, Family and Community Medicine, University of
Missouri/Columbia

This presentation of findings from the evaluation of joint practice is a deliberately selective compilation of project components deemed particularly relevant to the theme of this volume. The project sheds some light on the nature of the nursing presence in collaborative practice settings.

BACKGROUND

The effort to assess and evaluate joint practice–based care was first discussed with members of the staff of the W. K. Kellogg Foundation in 1979. Originally, the evaluation focused on the joint practice program that had been developed at the University of Missouri–Columbia in the context of an academically based primary family medicine and nurse practitioner training program. Subsequent discussions disclosed that it would be more advantageous theoretically and methodologically, as well as more useful to the foundation, to assess joint practice through a much greater scope of sampling and inquiry. Most of the joint practice programs supported by the W. K. Kellogg Foundation were included, and the focus of evaluation was broadened to include a wider range of characteristics of joint practice settings than the single issue of nurse practitioner and physician comparability. The project was initiated in 1981. It has succeeded in going beyond previously held perceptions and thus has provided an impetus for new questions and new directions of study. At the outset, several observations are in order to provide a focus on issues central to this study.

The difficulty of developing an appropriate, nonjudgmental, and rigorous methodology became self-evident as soon as we explored the existing literature. This examination of the literature showed that most previous studies of joint practice and of nurse practitioners had a flawed conceptual basis: almost all of them cast perceived patterns of physician behavior as the norms against which nurse practitioner performance was judged. This design not only prevented distinct nursing behaviors from being identified or described, but also failed to anchor physician behavior in any data-based criteria. Although some articles acknowledged that nurse practitioners apparently do some other things that are not identifiable in these research designs, and although many acknowledged that patients like these "other" activities, most authors dismissed these factors as insignificant because they did not correspond to physician behaviors. Clearly, a new project had to start from the very conceptual and methodological beginning in developing a research approach that did not predetermine occupationally linked attributes and norms.

In approaching this study and its findings, it is essential to look at both professions as distinct systems and distinct practice approaches. The persistent, and still prevailing assumption that the nurse practitioner in joint practice is essentially a substitute for a physician clouds the questions and distorts the findings. This glib and misleading view of joint practice, commonly held in medical circles and expressed in medical literature, is also espoused by a sizable segment of nursing. To view the nurse practitioner as a physician substitute hinders exploration of the nursing presence in joint practice. The project might indeed have produced data suggesting that the nurse practitioner is primarily an agent of physician care. Such a finding is only valid if the posing of the research design did not predetermine such results. It is a disservice to joint practice to start with the acceptance of a substitute role for the nurse practitioner when there has been no examination of the evidence. In fact, the careful methodology employed in the joint practice evaluation project discussed below revealed that, tradition and power notwithstanding, some nursing priorities distinct from medical behavior can be observed. To accept the relationship between nurse practitioners and physicians as complementary rather than subsidiary is a central theme of the research undertaken.

The project directors have spent many years working as researchers and teachers with nursing and medicine. On the basis of this experience, the thrust of the findings and many facets of the subcultures of the two professions could have been anticipated. Nevertheless, the blind wall of prejudice and stereotyping that both professions display toward the concept of copractice was a surprise. Neither profession was open to shedding light on this health care delivery experiment: leaders in both professions manifested intense hostility when joint practice was discussed. Some of the foremost thinkers in nursing categorically stated that there is no way in which a nurse can work closely with a physician without surrendering the essence of nursing. In some ways, it appears as if a battle has been declared lost before an engagement was ever risked. Likewise, a number of physicians, some in leadership positions, have asserted that there is absolutely no way of providing first-class care if a nurse practitioner is included as a caregiver. By definition, they argue, nurse practitioners provide second-class care.

It is noteworthy that the uncompromising, negative statements always came from individuals who either held offices in which they felt that they represented their respective profession or worked in practice settings that did not involve any present or past contact with collaborative opportunities. Those who are engaged in joint practice—i.e., those who formed the focal population for this study—hardly ever made such statements. The only negative comments came from those who were working through the first months of joint practice and thus were in a period of experimentation and adaptation. The great majority of those who were observed, whose stories were recorded, and whose behavior was videotaped—nurse practitioners and physicians alike—consistently acknowledge the value and benefits of cooperation for themselves and for their clients. They conveyed a strong sense of conviction that joint practice rests on preconditions of cooperation such as mutual respect and acceptance of the validity of their different perspectives.

To place our findings in the context of other data requires careful assessment of the conditions in which these data were generated. We consistently found that joint practice teams were aware of the negative attitudes of their respective peers and that their achieved level of collaboration frequently ran afoul of colleague pressures, formal procedures, and general expectations. Thus, studies of joint practice arrangements must be interpreted cautiously, since most of them do not operate under unfettered and unconstrained circumstances but rather have to be viewed as functioning under "closed closet" conditions. It was only when they could not be overheard and had made sure that they were alone with the researcher that several physicians in joint practice confided that after having worked several years with a nurse practitioner, they would again choose working with a nurse practitioner over the option of having a partnership with another physician. Usually, they added, "Don't ever expect me to say that at a meeting of the medical society."

Likewise, nurse practitioners, particularly in certain regions, meet their most serious obstacles in the reluctance of or refusal by nursing service administrators to accord the nurse practitioner practicing privileges in the local hospital. The most frequent reason given is that there is no "protocol for supervising" nurse practitioners. (The emphasis on the need for supervision documented in many studies of the nursing service organization has emerged in different studies as a focal point for real difficulties in creating conditions for genuine professional practice in institutional settings. It is contradictory for a profession to emphasize the autonomy and competence of the members and then insist on substantive supervision as a condition of employment.) Therefore, many nurse practitioners in that region resorted to the device of attaining licensure as a physician's assistant. In this way, practice privileges could be gained through the medical staff, with the department of nursing essentially having chased one of its own into an association and identification with the very profession from which nursing wishes to maintain a distinct identity.

The experiential (and subcultural) context of these data is crucially important, since it sheds light on the origin and meaning of the information gathered. This context provides some guidelines for establishing a baseline and a set of perimeters within which the data must be interpreted to enhance the understanding of the identified social realities. These data do not have a common point of neutral (or zero) value.

Although both members of the joint practice team function under surroundng constraints, the norms of joint practice do not have the same impact on physicians that they do on nurses. The medical identity, while taking into account the predominant medical norms and expectations, brings with it a sense of autonomy and self-assurance that reduces susceptibility to restraining messages. The long tradition of nursing, however, continues to carry significant remnants of subordination and subservience, and thus an orientation that values compliance with perceived or real physician norms. Consequently, the nurse practitioner in joint practice settings may be reluctant to display assertive and genuinely collegial behavior, even if the nurse practitioner's medical partner is ready for such a relationship. These internalized dimensions of restraint are linked not only with the traditions of the two professions but also with the simple fact that most physicians are male and most nurse practitioners female. Implications of the gender factor for professional identity will be discussed later as part of the study findings.

At this point, let it suffice to observe that the socialization of women in this society is still failing to incorporate assertiveness into the symbolic environment and the education of young women. Focusing on learned behaviors—e.g., preoccupation with the skills and techniques of assertiveness—is inadequate, because assertiveness becomes effective only when it is a comfortable component of a person's internalized behavior system. Thus, beneath the statements of belief and the description of arrangements, the physicians in the study tended to convey a much greater reliance on their own mode of operation than the nurse practitioner did. Having only recently established a distance between the role of the nurse practitioner and the compliant, humble tradition of nursing, nurse practitioners tended to feel more influenced by their perceived image of the physician's preferences than many of the physicians in the study actually expected them to. Even more suggestive for practice and education is our observation that the actual behavior captured with the help of the videotapes showed more indicators of a nursing presence and more identifiable reliance on a nursing model than the self-reports of the nurse practitioners and their charting would indicate.

Being involved in a project increases one's sensitivity to casual but relevant incidents. Just two days before the 1987 NLN Convention, one of us (H. M.) participated in a conference on science, technology, and the liberal arts. This conference was sponsored by the American Association for the Advancement of Science, and it brought together scholars and practitioners from a variety of fields. By chance, the coauthor was seated during the first lunch next to the only physician who was a participant in the conference. This physician serves as a part-time director of the medical education program at a well-known medical school and practices as a cardiac surgeon. In the course of conversation, the joint practice evaluation study was mentioned. The physician became visibly excited and showed great interest in the data and implications. He explained that he was experiencing ostracism and ridicule from other cardiac surgeons, who find it quite unacceptable that this surgeon works closely with a nurse practitioner as a partner. During the luncheon, the physician explained that he had discovered that the nurse practitioner could do things that had never been part of the medical repertory and that they could share with and learn from each other. He remarked, "She can run circles around me in preop and postop care, which makes it useful to work together and to listen to each other. All the other surgeons think that I am just going after fluff."

This has by no means been an isolated event. It is fascinating and suggestive that both authors have found themselves in a number of situations in which a physician, upon hearing about the joint practice evaluation study, "confidentially" shared his or her appreciation of joint practice and of nurse practitioners. At times, these statements have included views that would normally be considered radical and that place the contribution of the nurse practitioner to patient care on a level of value comparable to that of the work of the physician.

The organization of this paper to this point represents a departure from the usual organization of such reports. Whether these first pages are considered hors d'oeuvres or stage settings, we feel that it is important to provide an adequate background before presenting the actual data. The subtlety and complexity of the data are as much a result of the social context of the study as they are generic characteristics of the joint practice phenomenon per se. The design of the project involves the evaluation of the context of joint practice. Evaluation does not necessarily seek to test hypotheses; it may simply address certain questions. The following are some of the general research questions that have guided the project since the beginning.

1. Does joint practice provide patient care that in scope, quality, or client behavior differs from the care given by physicians or nurse practitioners alone?

2. Since joint practice as a concept is linked somewhat to the emergence of the nurse practitioner, does the nurse practitioner offer services that are distinct from those provided by a physician?
3. Does joint practice represent merely joining the two discreet health care roles, or does it involve modifications in the role and function of both participants?
4. Does joint practice offer tangible advantages that might make it more acceptable to the community of practitioners, who might otherwise perceive it as threatening, useless, or expensive, and can it be justified in the context of current consumer needs?

PROJECT STRUCTURE

The project itself is divided into three research phases. The first is an analytical examination of the literature that provides some basic support for trying to answer some of the research questions and aid in the design of methodologies. The literature also provides a database with the help of which certain kinds of research questions on the context of research being done on joint practice can be answered.

The second phase of the project involves a systematic data gathering process that centers on four foci: (1) the team, in particular its emergence, structure, and communication arrangements; (2) the team members, in particular the selection and suitability of professionals to enter joint practice settings; (3) the patient care outcome; and (4) the recognition and awareness of, as well as acceptance and response to, joint practice arrangements in various community segments under various conditions.

The third phase involves the development of a model for further evaluation of joint practice. Early in the history of the project, the research team confronted the need for a theoretical model that would be compatible with the project objectives and serve as a guide in the selection and development of the methodologies for data collection. On the basis of the four foci and the research questions, a preliminary theoretical model of the project was developed. This model had three sources. The first was a content analysis of explorator interviews with nurse practitioners and physicians in joint practice; the second was a content analysis of the literature on joint practice; and the third was an analysis of the basic issues in joint practice developed by the research team. The result of these analyses was a conceptual model or topography of joint practice.

The model begins with the abstract construct "joint practice" and partitions it into its constituents at increasingly concrete levels to arrive at the methodologies to be employed in data collection. The first division of the basic construct into three components that represent process, structure, and outcome forms the basis for the contextual description and evaluation of joint practice. The integration of structure, process, and outcome variables at the different levels of analysis provides a guide to the research design.

For example, the process of interactive behavior between patient and provider in joint practice involves the style of clinical interaction, which comprises specific statements from or characteristics of the clinic encounter. This process of delivering care in joint practice is then linked to the characteristics of the actors, the characteristics of the environment, and the patient care outcome.

PROJECT METHODS

The design of the empirical research phase meets the original goals and objectives of the project by being sensitive to the contextual factors that condition the delivery of health care in joint practice settings. The different methodologies used acknowledge the complexity of joint practice as a construct with many facets—e.g., behaviors of individuals, sets of norms, beliefs, and orientations. The methodologies were designed to maximize the provision of information about joint practice while minimizing the disruption of routine for the research subjects.

One of the key methodologies is the videotaping of a sample of provider–patient encounters. Use of these videotapes is necessary, since it is the only technique available that provides the researcher with comprehensive documentation of verbal, behavioral, and symbolic interactions (Erickson, 1982; Grimshaw, 1982; Duncan, 1982). It permits coding not only of tasks and content but also of the style and scope of a provider's work with the patient.

Brief interviews with the providers and the patients after these taped encounters gather data on the participants' point of view. Further details are obtained in a questionnaire that is distributed to providers. The questionnaire adds data on their personal orientations as well as on their priorities in caring for their patients. As part of the data collection, information is obtained on the various ways in which the collaborative team arranges the sharing and allocating of tasks and functions and how they arrange the organization of the joint practice. A brief follow-up telephone interview with providers and with the patients is scheduled about one month after the visit.

To date, the sample includes over 400 videotaped encounters with over 160 providers at approximately 60 sites located in different regions of the country. The encounters include a collection of well-care, acute, chronic, and follow-up visits that involve a wide variety of patients. The sites range from California to Philadelphia to eastern Kentucky to North Dakota. Since it is very difficult to obtain a representative sample when little information is available on how many joint practices really exist and on what, for example, the major mode of joint practice arrangements might be, the sample includes a variety of settings, from an urban practice to a small practice in a rural town of 1,500 people, from a health maintenance organization (HMO) to a major university. The settings are as diverse as the people that are participating in joint practice. There is not just one kind of joint practice arrangement but a plurality of arrangements.

As previously mentioned, one primary focus of the project was evaluating styles of interactive behavior during provider–patient encounters in the clinic. An observation methodology was developed to analyze providers' style of clinical interaction, which is a composite of interpersonal style and diagnostic/therapeutic style. Argyle (1972) has described style of interpersonal behavior as the set of characteristic techniques an actor employs to achieve certain goals or to solve certain kinds of problems. These techniques have both biological and cultural origins and are developed, adapted, and displayed according to the personal and interpersonal needs and experiences of the actors. The characteristic behavior a medical provider displays in dealing with patients can be viewed as a combination of personal and cultural qualities that are in some ways unique and in others typical of other providers in similar situations.

The clinical encounter is a specific type of interpersonal interaction that has both interpersonal and clinical goals. For example, the provider must be concerned both with maintaining patient cooperation and with making a proper clinical diagnosis. Thus, style of clinical interaction comprises both interpersonal style and diagnostic/therapeutic style.

The concept of interpersonal style has been addressed by a great number of writers (Argyle, 1972; Gough, 1957; Wiggins, 1982; Leary, 1957; Foa, 1961). The basic model of interpersonal style that emerges from the literature is a circumplex model (see Figure 1). The interpersonal style of an individual is measured as a function of behaviors exhibited along two dimensions: affiliation and control. Affiliative behaviors are those directed toward some form of intimacy with others (Argyle, 1972); control behaviors are those directed toward determining the course or outcome of the interaction.

The conceptual relationship between these dimensions of interpersonal style and the elements of diagnostic/therapeutic style is somewhat more complex (see Figure 2). The diagnostic/therapeutic dimensions of clinical style are those that are specific to the tasks that define patient care in the clinical setting. These dimensions are relevant to the clinical performance of both nurse practitioners and physicians and do not rest on the traditions and preferences of either profession.

Procedure

Provider–patient encounters were recorded by a videotape camera placed inside the examination room and positioned so that behaviors of both patients and providers were recorded. A video recorder was place in another room so that it could be controlled by the researchers in an unobtrusive manner. A lens cap was made available to the provider so that the camera lens could be covered during sensitive examinations in order to protect patient privacy. For each half-day of recording, one provider was selected, and arrangements were made with the staff to place that provider's patients in the taping room. Informed consent was obtained from each patient before taping.

A major advantage of using videotape was the freedom to review the tapes away from the clinical situation in order to refine the coding scheme used to analyze the interaction. There are two types of analysis of interaction: action analysis and content analysis (Duncan, 1982). Action analysis involves data on form; such as language, body movement, and paralanguage. Content analysis involves data on substance or meaning.

In the present study, analysis of observations was first approached from the action analysis perspective. It soon became apparent, however, that this type of analysis was too atomistic to be useful in the study of certain aspects of clinical interaction. Inui, Carter, Kukull, and Haigh (1982) reached the same conclusion in a study of doctor–patient interaction, namely, that action analysis systems were not the best methods for the study of clinical encounters at a relatively holistic level. Action analysis of provider–patient interaction was not abandoned in the present study, however; rather, it was supplemented by a content analysis designed to measure the style of providers. The action analysis methodology was used to supplement the data on affiliation and control in the interpersonal style measurement and was the primary source of data on communication strategies.

Since this study includes both physicians and nurse practitioners, it was important that the content analysis encompass aspects of both physician and nurse practitioner roles. Bibb (1982) found in a study of nurse practitioners and physicians that the main difference between these providers was the inclusion by nurse practitioners of expressive "caring" functions, such as health education, more extensive follow-up and explanation, discussion of prevention, inclusion of support and comfort measures in treatment plans, identification of psychosocial factors, and use of community resources. These functions were, therefore, included in the present content analysis, along with other functions ostensibly more typical of the medical role. A coding form was developed by the team, tested, reviewed, and modified until consensus was reached on the categories to be coded. An attempt was made to provide examples that could be used to distinguish between very similar categories in order to reduce the ambiguity inherent in this type of analysis. The coding scheme was reviewed by physician and nurse practitioner consultants. Their suggestions were considered, and appropriate adaptations were made.

The coding process itself involved recording the number of statements made or questions asked by the provider about the particular content area. The categories on the coding form represented numbers of statements. For example, how often did the person talk about the chronology of the illness? (One statement, two statements, three statements, or more.) This approach not only described what was done, but also suggested the intensity with which it was done. Scores for individual items on the coding form were then combined to form indices of the components of clinical interaction style.

Since a provider's score on any of the observational indices is affected by the length of the patient encounter, the scores were corrected for this by expression of each one as a proportion of the total number of activities coded for the encounter. Utilizing the same episodes, reliability calculations for this type of analysis have demonstrated intrarater and interrater reliabilities of greater than 80 percent.

The action analysis of the encounters involved coding verbal utterances on 28 different criteria and was designed to evaluate communication strategies. Together, the observation analyses took about seven hours to code 15 minutes of interaction.

FINDINGS

Preliminary findings on attitudes toward joint practice indicate that familiarity breeds acceptance and appreciation. Physicians who had direct contact with nurse practitioners in academic or private joint practice proved to be aware of the benefits associated with joint practice. Most of them readily acknowledged respect for the areas of competence of nurse practitioners and for their special contributions to the clinic. Conversely, physicians without direct experience with nurse practitioners were much more likely to display negative attitudes and to base their rejection on stereotypes. It is interesting to note that, to judge from statements by physicians who work with nurses in traditional hierarchical relationships, such relationships with nurses were not linked to a greater acceptance of nurse practitioners.

Patients generally accepted joint practice arrangements, were able to identify the nurse practioner role, and had predominantly positive orientations toward that role. Yet a real understanding of the nurse practitioner and an awareness of all the implications of joint practice could not be identified in patient responses. This observation may be partly linked to the general lack of analytic approaches shown by clients of professional services, but it may also be linked to the actual experiences of patients. The data indicate that in day-to-day clinical interaction, the behavior of physicians and nurse practitioners showed only a few subtle differences.

Preliminary findings on styles of clinical interaction seem to support this observation: there was very little variation in interpersonal style among providers. Providers tend to do the same kind of things for the same kind of visit. In fact, nurse practitioners and physicians varied their affiliative and control behavior for different types of visits and visit histories in similar ways. A discriminant analysis showed that the two variables that discriminated most effectively in terms of interpersonal behavior were type of visit and visit history. Thus, both nurse practitioners and physicians varied their actions according to whether a visit was a first, second, or third or later one and according to whether it was an acute, a well, a chronic, or a follow-up one.

Although there were few differences between the styles of nurse practitioners and physicians when all visits were considered together, an interesting difference between nurse practitioners and physicians emerged when type of visit was controlled for. Nurse practitioners did have higher mean scores than physicians on this dimension, but only on well-care visits did nurse practitioners show significantly greater psychosocial concern than physicians. Given the psychosocial emphasis in nurse practitioner training and nurses' preference for and perceived proficiency in this area, one would expect to find more instances of increased concern for psychosocial issues on the part of nurse practitioners. This finding was interesting, since the data indicate that it only occurred in visits that were not focused on illness phenomena. Apparently, prevailing patterns of behavior and the current organization of work still emphasize traditional medical concerns; many nurse practitoners still followed a medical behavior model, despite their preferences and areas of competence. As mentioned earlier, tradition, power, and risk avoidance make the medical model appear safe. The ideals expressed by nurse practitioners differed from the behavior actually observed and from the information entered in the chart.

The effect of a specific illness focus on provider behavior was also shown by the finding that provider sensitivity in general, and sensitivity associated with the physical examination in particular, were highest for well-care visits and lowest for acute and follow-up visits. In well-care visits, providers do not need to focus on a specific illness state. This allows them greater freedom in the interaction and more time for relationship development.

There were only a few differences in provider sensitivity toward the patient between nurse practitioners and physicians in joint practice, but they both displayed more sensitivity than physicians in solo practice. Physicians in joint practice were apparently more like the partner they worked with than they were like physicians in solo practice. Thus, there is some evidence that there is a shift from professional independence to professional interdependence within a joint practice. This observation suggests a nursing approach can exert considerable influence on a physician, provided that there is an acceptance of complementarity and mutual respect.

Another difference in provider behavior related to type of visit was the greater number of support- and comfort-related behaviors in visits for chronic problems. By definition, a chronic problem is one for which there is no immediately curative intervention; supportive measures may be the only resource available to alleviate patients' discomfort or improve their functioning. By this same reasoning, one would expect to find use of support/comfort measures to be lowest for acute visits, in which curative interventions would be the focus. This was indeed the case in the present study.

Providers were also found to vary their clinical style for different patient age groups. In general, older patients have more chronic or severe problems related to illness and general dysfunction. With older patients, providers exhibited styles that emphasized history taking, diagnostic/therapeutic activity, and psychosocial concern. Older patients were also likely to have been seeing the same primary care provider for a long time, which contributed to greater patient and provider comfort. This was shown by higher patient-perceived sensitivity, provider affiliation, and patient control in these visits.

Findings for clinical interaction style when visit history was controlled for reveal changes in both provider and patient behaviors over time. Provider behavior was higher in psychosocial concern, history taking, physical examination activity, affiliation, and control in first or second visits, and significantly lower in these activities in third or subsequent visits. These findings reflect the process of getting-to-know the patient in a physical and socioemotional sense and building a comfortable relationship. Patient behavior was lower in affiliation and control in first and second visits and significantly higher after the second visit. This indicates increasing comfort with the relationship, demonstrated by friendlier, more autonomous patient behavior.

Providers were more affiliative with female patients, and female patients were more affiliative with providers than male patients were and perceived more psychosocial concern. Overall, female patients tended to be much more sensitive to the psychosocial dimensions present in the interaction than male patients were. The highest affiliation was between male providers and female patients; the lowest was between male providers and male patients.

Preliminary findings also indicate that there were differences in how patients behaved toward physicians and how they behaved toward nurse practitioners. Patient control was higher with physicians than with nurse practitioners in chronic and follow-up visits and higher with nurse practitioners than with physicians in well-care visits. Patient affiliation was higher with physicians in all visit history categories and all types of visit categories except for acute visits, in which affiliation levels for physicians and nurse practitioners were the same. Although patients in a joint practice usually see both the physician and the nurse practitioner, they may consider the physician to be the authority figure and feel that it is more important to develop a good relationship with the physician. The reversal of this pattern for well-care visits may indicate that patients perceive this type of visit to be the province of the nurse practitioner. Physicians also may be perceived to have higher status than nurse practitioners; if so, patients logically would want to be liked by the higher status provider as well as to maintain their autonomy in the relationship.

High patient affiliation/high patient control coupled with high provider affiliation/low provider control resulted in higher patient satisfaction than any other combination of patient and provider interaction styles. This combination was also associated with low history taking, higher patient participation, and high provider sensitivity as perceived by the patient. The data also indicate that patient satisfaction was influenced more by patient perceptions than by the actual events that occurred during a clinical encounter.

Patient satisfaction is only one of many outcome measures. Patient compliance is another that is frequently studied. One important factor affecting compliance is patient recall of information, instructions, or recommendations. In this context, the results of this study are encouraging for joint practice. Patients who saw a nurse practitioner or who were seen by both a nurse practitioner and a physician recalled significantly more information on follow-up than patients seen in a solo practice. Although recall does not ensure patient performance of suggested activities, failure to recall instructions make performance unlikely. Patients who perceived greater information provision recalled more information on follow-up, regardless of the actual amount of information presented.

The data on provider satisfaction with various tasks and their perceived proficiency in performing these tasks showed that nurse practitioners expressed greater satisfaction with patient education, psychosocial assessments, preventive teaching, guidance, and counseling activities and felt more proficient in these areas. Physicians reported greater satisfaction with activities related to diagnosis and treatment and claimed greater proficiency in these activities.

The gender segregation within the health professions, with nurse practitioners being predominantly female and physicians being predominantly male, could result in difficulties in joint practice relationships that reflect the gender struggles in the larger society. The results of this study suggest that gender-related influences on joint practice teams may be less than anticipated. Male and female providers displayed similar clinical interaction styles, and patients were equally satisfied with male and female providers.

As an adjunct methodology, a sample of providers were shown four videotaped patient–provider clinical encounters involving a male physician, a male nurse practitioner, a female physician, and a female nurse practitoner. When asked to identify the status of the provider in each episode, these providers associated the professional roles of nurse practitioner and physician with female and male gender, respectively. Respondents who viewed a female provider assumed that she was a nurse practitioner, and respondents who viewed a male provider assumed that he was a physician. This stereotypical attribution occurred even though the clinical behavior of the female physician was more like that of the male physician than like that of the female nurse practitioner. Likewise, the clinical behavior of the male nurse practitioner was more like that of the female nurse practitioner than like that of the male physician.

The current findings of the joint practice evaluation project emphasize the complexity of the factors affecting cooperative practice between physicians and nurse practitioners. Although the data collected and analyzed after three years of research have to be viewed as reports of an ongoing study, several findings warrant a reassessment of approaches to the evaluation of joint practice arrangements. Stereotypes of gender and occupation, inequality of status and power, and actual distribution of gender were factors in analyzing the processes and products of joint practice arrangements. Yet these variables, though important, proved to be less powerful than was anticipated. Detailed analysis yielded fewer clear distinctions between nurse practitioners and physicians than might have been expected. The factor that emerged as a major force in the functioning of joint practice teams turned out to be the persistance of the traditional medical model. This model not only restrained nurse practitioners from practicing or recording behaviors derived from a nursing model, but also influenced the behavior of physicians, who seemed to feel pressure against expanding into broader approaches to patient care. Thus, while in some instances the complementarity of nurse practitioner and physician approaches ran into problems stemming from unequal power, both team members were more typically controlled by the weight of medical tradition.

RESPONSES AND IMPLICATIONS

These findings evoke a number of responses. First and foremost, the importance and implications of the subtlety of these data has to be reemphasized. Neither assumptions of normal distribution nor assumptions of free and unskewed reporting of information can be applied to this harvest of observations, self-reports, and questionnaire responses. No matter how slight the differences, attention should be paid to the indicators that show that, regardless of gender, physicians and nurse practitioners reflect their respective occupation when their actual behavior is examined, but perceptions of them, whether by professional peers or by the public, is dominated by gender stereotypes. This point has far-reaching implications for practice, for professional education, and for media management.

At the same time, one can respond to the findings as being largely expectable and containing no major surprises. What is probably the most difficult aspect of this study to document, yet possibly the most significant aspect in the long term, is the accumulated cues that something occurs in joint practice that may not be fully captured even by the careful methdology thought to be adquate for this project. The suggestion that in some ways physicians and nurse practitioners in joint practice seem to absorb some of each other's style and behaviors appears to contradict the impression that the collaborative arrangement actually frees each partner to be more of a physician, or more of a nurse practitioner. In fact, both are probably true, paradoxic though it may seem. The collaborative model may indeed offer the nurse practitioner a better opportunity to demonstrate a nursing presence and to implement a nursing model of care than traditional institutional settings, where constraints and pressures give higher priority to medical and managerial activities then to the core of nursing.

Another dimension not immediately identifiable from the systematically assembled data was the relationship within the team. Observations, casual remarks, and the physical and social context of the clinics visited provided a fairly adequate picture of the degree to which the term "joint practice" was an operational reality rather than merely a label. We did find many settings in which complementary and collegial relationships were the prevailing pattern, but we also found many that under the guise of collaborative practice retained strong remnants of traditional physician–nurse structures. The importance of not only mutual respect but also the acceptance of different priorities and styles emerged as a key ingredient of a successful joint practice team. It was under these conditions that mutual learning was a free exchange among colleagues rather than the mere emulation of a more powerful model.

There is potentially far-reaching significance to the finding that physicians in joint practice differ noticeably from physicians who work in clinics in which no involvement of nurse practitioners and other nurses is the pattern. It is fascinating to contemplate the implications of the findings that acceptance, respect, and partnership serve as the lubricant for adoptive behavior and for learning. Physicians in joint practice not only manifested changes due to the nursing presence but actually acknowledge them. There is no evidence that physicians working with nurses in traditional subordinate positions were in any way affected by the behaviors and practice style of these nurses. In many cases, they probably did not even notice them.

The characteristics of the joint practice setting varied as a result of differences in individual practices and of factors introduced through individual personalities and preferences. It should not be forgotten, however, that some collective factors are at work and that local cultures, region, and the climate set by the respective medical and nursing schools influenced the readiness for collaborative relationships. The physical layout of the clinic and offices, although beyond the control of the team itself, was found to be of great importance. Office facilities that were identical in location, size, and furnishings for nurse practitioners and physicians alike were most consistently found in practices located in California, north of Sacramento. In that region, it was also observed that the listings in the Yellow Pages give the names and titles of the physician and the nurse practitioner equal prominence and size. In a very different vein, we were impressed that in the family practice clinics located in some of the most desperately underserved areas of the Bronx, the urgency of the situation, the dramatic needs being met, and the commitment of all staff members minimized, if not eliminated, status differences, status prerogatives, and traditional allocation of tasks.

An important dimension of the cultural context could be observed in North Dakota and in southern California. Both of these areas have strong ethnic concentrations, and nurse practitioners were more likely to be of the local ethnic group than physicians were. This not only placed nurse practitioners in the position of occasional translators, but also, more subtly, made them legitimating agents whose advice was sought about the acceptability of the physicians.

The thrust of the project findings should be placed in its proper perspective. Researchers are committed to examine any social phenomenon fairly. Thus, whatever the results, we do not act as advocates for joint practice. Both participant professions are treated with respect. The focus of this inquiry is the identification of factors that influence the delivery of joint practice–based care. A further aim of this project is to show that joint practice should be given a fair opportunity to be demonstrated and evaluated. It is time for both professions, particularly the leaders, to reconsider their negative judgment about collaborative arrangements and respond to this innovative approach to family health care without hiding behind a wall of stereotypes. All human beings need respect and recognition from others. A successful joint practice team is usually based on a relationship of respect and acceptance. This is lacking in contacts with those of colleagues who look at joint practice as some form of betrayal. The overall theme of this project underscores the need nurse practitioners and physicians have for recognition and support. Joint practices in the United States are in hiding from the negative pressure emanating from their respective peers and by so doing keep the door of the closet closed. This admonition is particularly relevant to nursing, where a climate of colleagueship, pride, and mutual support is desperately needed.

Although this report contains a considerable amount of suggestive insights and data, it is important to remember that at this time our data are still preliminary and thus must be considered tentative until data analysis is completed.

The implications of this project are not limited to options in the structure of primary care and to issues of communications between nursing and medicine. The study has potentially significant implications for the education of nurse practitioners and physicians. Better understanding of the structure and function of other health professions and respect for diverse roads leading to the same helping goal should be part of the medical and nursing school curriculum. Joint practice relationships do not emerge out of a formal set of aggreements; rather, they rely on early socialization as youths and as professionals to set the stage that will enable the two providers to join in the effort to develop a team.

This condition applies to both professions, but there is an additional dimension that the nursing programs must face. Although the number of males in nursing has increased slightly, nursing is still primarily a profession of women. To relate to someone who is usually older, male, and prestigious requires a firmly internalized sense of worth and the ability to be comfortably assertive. It has to be recognized and addressed that a proclivity to subservience and uncertainty about oneself is not primarily due to personality; in fact, its manifestation is based on historical facts. The very upbringing of young males and females, even in the 1980s, is quite distinct. Like all minority groups, women, and in this case nurses, have internalized a lack of confidence in themselves. Most tragic of all, the nursing profession, like other minority groups, demonstrates that members of a systematically undervalued group are bound to internalize some of these messages and consequently to encounter difficulty in feeling respect and loyalty for others in the same group. Schools of nursing must recognize that assertiveness skills cannot be adequately taught in formal, cognitive skill-oriented courses. The acquisition of assertiveness touches the very inner regions of those we wish to help to become assertive. The implication of this project suggest strongly that the most thorough and scholarly educational preparation for professional nursing may never be put into practice unless the educational institutions address the needs and role shifts of the person who is in the process of becoming a nurse.

The two principal investigators have learned immeasurably from the study and from each other. The differences in their own scientific and methodologic backgrounds have provided an opportunity for truly collaborative research practices. The result was a genuinely triangulated design that expresses respect for the pluralistic characteristics of the data and for the need to tap social reality from several vantage points.

REFERENCES

Argyle, M. (1972). *The psychology of interpersonal behavior* (2nd ed.). London: Cox and Wyman.

Bibb, B. N. (1982). Comparing nurse practitioners and physicians: A simulation study on processes of care. *Evaluation and the health professions, 5* (1), 29–42.

Brent, E. E., Jr. (1979). Patient-practitioner interaction in the medical history interview: An empirical test of a Markov model. Unpublished manuscript, University of Missouri.

Corley, M. C., Mauksch, H. O. (1987). *Registered nurses, gender, and commitment.* In A. Statham, E. Miller, & H. O. Mauksch (Eds.). *The value of women's work: Qualitative approaches.* Albany, NY: SUNY University Press.

Duncan, S., Jr. (1982). Quantitative studies of interaction structure and strategy. *Sociological Methods and Research, 2* (2), 175–194.

Erickson, F. (1982). Audiovisual records as a primary data source. *Sociological Methods and Research, 2* (2), 213–232.

Foa, U. G. (1961). Convergences in the analysis of the structure of interpersonal behavior. *Psychological Review, 68,* 341–353.

Gordon, L. V. (1976). *Survey of interpersonal values: Revised manual.* Chicago: Science Research Associates.

Gough, H. G. (1957). *Manual for the California Psychological Inventory.* Palo Alto, CA: Consulting Psychologists Press.

Grimshaw, A. D. (1982). Sound-image data records for research on social interaction: Some questions and answers. *Sociological Methods and Research, 2* (2), 121–144.

Harper, P. (1985). Joint practice: A selected annotated bibliography. New York: Garland.

Inui, T. S., Carter, W. B., Kukull, W. A., & Haigh, V. H. Outcome-based doctor–patient interaction analysis: I. Comparison of techniques. *Med Care, 20* (6), 535–566.

Leary, T. (1957). Interpersonal diagnosis of personality. New York: Ronald Press.

Mauksch, H. O., Campbell, J. D. (1985). Political imperatives for nursing in a stereotyping world. *Perspectives in nursing, 1985 – 1987.* New York: National League for Nursing.

Megargee, E. I. (1982). *The California Psychological Inventory handbook.* San Francisco: Jossey-Bass.

Stiles, W. B. (1978). Verbal response modes and dimensions of interpersonal roles: A method of discourse analysis. *Journal of Personality and Social Psychology, 36,* 693–703.

Wiggins, J. S. (1982). Circumplex models of interpersonal behavior in clinical psychology. In P. C. Kendall and J. M. Butcher (Eds.). *Handbook of Research Methods in Clinical Psychology* (pp. 183–221). New York: John Wiley and Sons.

ACKNOWLEDGMENTS

We are indebted to W. K. Kellogg Foundation for accepting and generously supporting the very expensive methodology used, which was based on videotaping sample encounters and subjecting these tapes to exhaustive analysis. After this experience, we would consider the absence of this record of real behavior as a serious flaw in a study design.

Figure 1. Model of Interpersonal Style

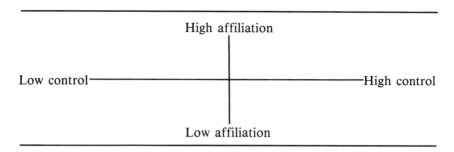

Figure 2. Model of Style of Clinical Interaction

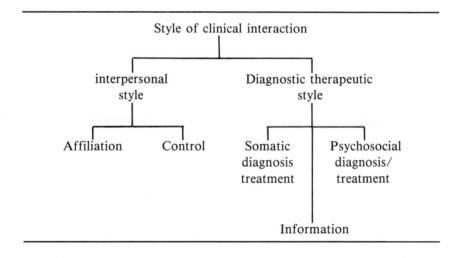

EDUCATING NURSE ADMINISTRATORS IN LONG-TERM CARE IN A CHANGING ENVIRONMENT

Carol Reed Ash, EdD, RN, FAAN
Associate Dean, Continuing Education
Marion A. Buckley School of Nursing
Adelphi University
Garden City, NY

Mary P. Lodge, EdD, RN
Director
Professional Education and Practice of Nurse Administrators/
Directors of Nursing in Long-Term Care Project
American Nurses' Foundation
Kansas City, MO

Helen Yura, PhD, RN, FAAN
Eminent Professor of Nursing and Graduate Program Director
School of Nursing
College of Health Services
Old Dominion University, Norfolk, VA

PHASE I

The long-term care project that we will be describing in this chapter was in operation for six years. It was terminated as of December 1987, but as we look forward to the decade ahead, it seems likely that work on long-term care is just beginning.

Phase I of this project, entitled "Professional Practice for Nurse Administrators in Long-Term Care Facilities," was conducted from May 1, 1981, through April 30, 1984. It was partially funded by the W. K. Kellogg Foundation of Battle Creek, Michigan, and cosponsored by the American College of Health Care Administrators, with Dr. Robert Burmeister as one

177

codirector, and by the American Nurses' Foundation, with one of us (M.P.L.) as the other codirector. Some 80 individuals from nursing in long-term care participated in this project over its years of operation. The work has been done through various committees of the project. Each of the outcomes and recommendations has come from committee action, collaborative action by representatives from long-term care, and action on the part of corporations and consumer organizations interested in long-term care. We have had in the project representatives of the National League for Nursing, the American Nurses' Association (which, for course, is the mother organization of the American Nurses' Foundation), and the American Association of Colleges of Nursing.

Phase I included the first national survey of nurse administrators in long-term care in the United States; some of the findings will be addressed later. As a result of this survey, we set up a task force to develop a new and comprehensive statement of the roles, responsibilities, and qualifications for nurse administrators in long-term care. This statement also was accompanied by curriculum implications, general topics that might be addressed in order to arrive at an understanding of the roles and responsibilities. The task force used the national survey results as well as their own experiences. We also asked the School of Nursing at Hunter College (of the City University of New York), the Brookdale Center for Aging of Hunter College, and the Mount Sinai Medical School of Medicine–Hunter College Long-Term Care Gerontology Center to develop for us, under contract, a paper that would outline the history of nursing administration in long-term care, including the role and responsibilities of the nurse administrator, and would also direct us to the 21st century. What would the needs of the aged be then, and what would be the role and responsibility of the nurse administrator in long-term care?

The task force had representatives from nursing, from long-term care, and from consumer organizations, such as the American Association for Retired Persons and the National Coalition for Nursing Home Reform. We also had representatives from Beverly Enterprises, which is one of the largest of the long-term care corporations in the United States, and the Hillhaven Corporation. We had input from the long-term care field all the way. The American Health Care Association—the largest of the long-term care organizations in the United States, with some 8,000 agency members—the American Association of Homes for the Aging, and the American College of Health Care Administrators were more fully represented in the second and third phases.

In the first phase, we went on to develop the continuing education program, which had a self-assessment inventory, faculty advisement and career counseling, with a series of self-instructional curriculum clusters/modules. All of these evolved from the statement of roles, responsibilities, and qualifications. We then wrote recommendations for Phase I.

PHASE II

In phase II of the project, we changed the title to "Professional Education and Practice of Nurse Administrators/Directors of Nursing in Long-Term Care." (We found that we had to accompany the title of nurse administrator with that of director of nursing; this was a result of our advisory committee recommendation in the first part of the project.) Phase II was sponsored solely by the American Nurses' Foundation and partially funded by the Kellogg Foundation. During phase II, which lasted from July 1984 until April 1986, selected universities began to implement the continuing education program. We planned with these universities for several years before implementing the program. Eight universities were selected: Adelphi University, Garden City, New York; Rush University, Chicago, Illinois; the University of Texas at Arlington; Indiana University, Indianapolis; University of Kansas, Kansas City, Kansas; Old Dominion University, Norfolk, Virginia; Ohio State University, Cleveland; and Louisiana State University, New Orleans. The development and implementation work that these faculty accomplished is worth a history in itself.

Phase II continued the work of dissemination. During that phase, we wrote a book on phase I (Lodge, 1985) and initiated additional alliances with the long-term care field. We had alliances through the phase I advisory committee, but we began to develop others and reach out to the long-term care industry to a greater degree. We were convinced that we had to have people in long-term care who had influence, who knew their organizations, because we had been advised, in an informal meeting, that we should start at the top and meet people, and then gradually we would come to know others and understand what needed to be done. In light of this, the new alliances were very important. It took a good deal of time, travel, and discussion to secure the initial representatives. It was interesting that in phase III, when we asked for continuing representation, we had no difficulty obtaining it. By then, we knew the people and they knew us, and we had built up between us a certain degree of confidence and trust.

In phase II, then, we completed the book, made new alliances, and went on to develop a manual of incentives and support mechanisms. We had to sell this program, so we decided to have the long-term care industry and nursing work together to build the manual. Meetings of a committee of national long-term care executives and nurses, followed by different meetings with regional representatives, were held twice in regions across the United States; thus, we had major input from all over the United States into our manual of incentives and support mechanisms. This manual is presented in the book we later wrote on phase II (Lodge & Pietraschke, 1986). Once again, several recommendations came out of phase II.

PHASE III

The third phase of the project lasted from May 1, 1986, to December 31, 1987. During this phase, one of us (M.P.L.) moved from ANA headquarters in Kansas City to the department of nursing education at Teachers College, Columbia University. The work of the project also moved from a full-time basis to a part-time one. The ANA had had its representatives in each of the project phases; however, in this phase we asked for representatives from the Cabinet on Nursing Education, the Cabinet on Nursing Practice, the Cabinet on Nursing Service, and the Council on Gerontological Nursing, because they were the groups that could be involved in leading and spearheading this work.

Over the years, the American Nurses' Foundation and the American Nurses' Association have maintained an excellent working knowledge of the work and concerns of this project, and we believe that some of the ANA House of Delegate recommendations have been an outgrowth of project effort. Nursing in long-term care is now one of the priorities of the American Nurses' Association. The project recommended that there be a National Commission on Long-Term Care Nursing (phase II); this recommendation has been supported by the ANA House of Delegates. Another recommendation out of the project (phase II) was that a magnet study of nursing homes be conducted. Our colleagues in the National League for Nursing have also worked side-by-side with us in the project, and we have been kept informed of their work related to long-term care, their position statements, and their publications.

A major goal of phase III was not to let the recommendations from phases I and II stay on paper or on the shelf. Representatives met three times during this phase with all representatives continuing from the other phases, as well as with the new ANA group just mentioned. We asked them "to suggest the ways and means that you feel your organization or the entity that you represent can use to implement and move forward the recommendations and outcomes of phases I and II of the project." At this point, we have a great deal of material, which we are analyzing and preparing for publication. We have also presented the project at meetings and conferences. We have written for the first time in *The Provider,* the American Health Care Association's official organ. To be able to explain our project and the import of it to the long-term care industry from a nursing education point of view was a landmark achievement. We are certain that the long-term care industry has a role alongside nursing in the decade ahead in improving long-term nursing care.

The performance of the cooperating universities has been remarkable, especially considering that they had to get their own funds and had to plan and figure out their approaches. They had our packet of materials. We were linked with them in site visits, in discussion of problems and concerns, and in development of needed materials. The institutions really turned themselves inside out to get the nurse administrators to the continuing education program. Over 500 nurse administrators took the self-assessment inventory; however, there is quite a discrepancy between those who took the self-assessment and those who enrolled in the curriculum cluster series in the continuing education program. Over 100 people took one or two of the curriculum clusters/modules, and ten people finished the requirements that they agreed on with faculty. In the meantime, what we are doing is starting an entity. We're learning, we're writing, and we're sharing, and we hope that this will help others in the future.

CONTINUING EDUCATION PROGRAM

As mentioned earlier, there was a national survey of the nurse administrators, and one of the elements surveyed was the continuing education preferences for the nurse administrators. As a result of the data that were obtained, over 2,500 problems and topics were suggested. Results of the analysis of this material indicates interest in the following subject areas: These were clinical nursing management–which comprised about 33 percent of the topical areas, and then the rest, which comprised more than 65 percent and had to do with such areas as department management and supervision, administrative skills, and human resource management. The other piece of the foundation for the continuing education program is the statement of roles, responsibilities, and qualifications. Out of that came areas of focus, such as organizational management, human resource management in nursing, nursing and health services management, and professional nursing and long-term care leadership.

This was the framework within which the continuing education program was developed by participants, with one of us (N.Y.) heading the self-instructional curriculum modules effort. We did not have free rein to do what we would have liked to do; we were constrained by the outcomes from the project. Thus, the program consists of three major areas, the first of which is the self-assessment development process, which has as a core element the self-assessment inventory. This inventory was developed by a committee comprising leaders and practitioners in nursing; there was also representation from nursing education, nursing administration, and long-term care. This group worked very diligently to develop, pilot test, update, revise, and improve the series of questions that make up the inventory. The final inventory had 120 questions that would be typical of the experience of the nurse administrator in long-term care.

The whole idea behind self-assessment was that it would be prescriptive. It was called an inventory instead of a test, so that the nurse administrator would have some sense of his or her strengths and areas needing improvement. In a sense, it combined assessment with education, and it served as a first step and encouraged an enhancement of professional growth and the achievement of excellence. The aim of the process itself was to assess participants' knowledge and skill level and also to help them make some informed career decisions for themselves. The content grew right out of the preliminary data from the project. Basically, it was not meant to be used by itself: it was to be used with the other two components of the program.

The second component of the program was the career counseling process, the purpose of which was to designate a faculty member from one of the cooperating universities with the nurse administrator in long-term care to review the results of the self-assessment inventory. This was to be an interactional, collaborative effort, so that strengths and limitations could be diagnosed. In addition, there was a discussion about career options. Many of the directors of nursing had no idea about some of the career options avilable. More than 70 percent of these people had the diploma in nursing as their highest educational experience; these were introduced to the baccalaureate degree in nursing as an educational option, and those few who had the baccalaureate degree in nursing were introduced to the master's degree in nursing. Part of the qualifications contained in the statement indicated that the baccalaureate degree in nursing was required now and that by 1990 or 1992 the master's degree in nursing, with preparation for administration and long-term care, would be the expectation. In addition to the formalized university education, nursing administrators were introduced to the varied continuing education courses and programs available, and particularly this one which was developed precisely for this group and was intended to be a stopgap-type program that would help improve the practice of the nurse administrator right away. They were also introduced to the certification process for nurse administrators through the ANA and helped to make some career plans for themselves on the basis of their own stated objectives. For some, this was their first experience with thinking about their future over the next five or ten years. Follow-up counseling sessions were established, which in many instances became an enriching experience for the nurse administrator in long-term care, who often had no one to talk with.

The third portion of the continuing education program was the self-instructional curriculum clusters/modules. These also were developed by a committee of nurses from nursing education, nursing administration, long-term care, and gerontologic nursing; there were also representatives of nursing organizations. In the end, there were six self-instructional clusters containing 31 modules in all. The clusters and the modules actually complemented the inventory, and the scoring complemented the modules, so that if there was a limitation in a particular area, it would point directly to the cluster and the modules that were the means to offset that particular deficiency. The clusters had to be taken as a whole. It was not necessary to take all six of them—some took only one or two—but none of them could be broken up; that is, a participant could not just take one or two modules and consider that sufficient. The first cluster was entitled "Institutional Organization and Administration"; the second, "Development, Implementation, and Evaluation of the Nursing Service Department"; the third, "Interrelationships, Research, Education and Service"; the fourth, "Human Resources Management"; the fifth, "System of Nursing Care Delivery"; and the sixth, "Enhancing the Nursing Knowledge Base for Directors of Nursing/Nurse Administrators in Long-Term Care." Between them, the six clusters spanned a considerable area for advancement through continuing education for the nurse administrator.

Certain recommendations and strategies came as a result of pilot testing these particular clusters and modules on a regional basis. There was some revision and updating of some of the references; there were references that were required and references that were optional, as there were learning experiences that were required and learning experiences that were optional. The revisions were made, and they finished final testing in December. Sometime soon, this whole continuing education program package will be prepared for sale to interested persons who would be involved in enhancing nurse administrators' experience in long-term care.

A few points about the program may need clarification. A cluster is defined as a set of instructional modules that are interrelated and together meet a very specific goal. It is made clear throughout the whole package that a module is a set of learning experiences intended to facilitate the learners' achievement and the demonstration of an objective. Although this is a self-instructional experience, the nurse administrator does have a faculty member who serves as advisor and is available as needed. In many instances, this faculty advisor turned out to be a significant support system for the nurse administrator, and some very important problem-solving was accomplished that benefited the nurse administrator on the job. The particular cluster/module design included the title, the rationale, and the clusters; each cluster also had a rationale, objectives, and the modules; and each of the modules had a rationale, intended learning outcomes, prerequisites, learning activities, optional learning activities, a post-test, and a bibliography. We hope that this package will become an ever more common sight in the future.

IMPLEMENTATION

It remains to be seen how we are going to implement this material and we are going to encourage people to come to the universities. The program was originally launched, or intended to be launched, by the eight universities in the fall of 1983, when, with some funding from the original sources, each university agreed to hold a conference and to invite organizations from the immediate area (150- to 200-mile radius) to come to the program for the purposes of finding out what the self-assessment process was all about, assessing the managerial skills of the people who came to it, describing the professional development opportunities that there were in nursing, and identifying the elements in the self-instructional curriculum modular approach to learning. Obviously, it was also an attempt to get these people to examine a curriculum cluster module, because the strategy was to improve the nursing administration of these people in long-term care facilities through this kind of approach. It is important to point out that initially only four of the eight programs planned were in fact conducted, because of a small response. We point that out because as the universities worked to get the information out there, it was very clear that that was a catalyst; as people became more aware of what was happening, response improved.

So the role of the university was clearly to deal with the self-assessment process, the faculty advisement and career counseling, and to offer the self-instructional curriculum clusters and modules. The universities did not in fact have any money for this, which indicates that the cooperating universities involved in this role were involved because they were really committed and felt the need to provide this kind of information to the long-term care people and to nursing administrators. The universities used different approaches; the majority put together advisory committees or steering committees, which for the most part were multidisciplinary so as to involve people who were in key positions in the long-term care industry and people who might be in a position to provide financial support for either people or faculty.

We believe that the multidisciplinary committees did a great deal to get the information to the targeted audiences. The advertising that was used took on many forms, depending on the dollars that the different cooperating universities had to put forth—special flyers, ongoing catalogues, introductory workshops, newsletters; many of the universities sent people out to meet with consumer groups and professional groups in long-term care. Individual letters and telephone calls were used to follow up the inquiries that came in when people found out what was going on. Eventually, the response became overwhelming. That the information would precipitate 30, 40 or 50 calls in a relatively small regional area illustrates that there was in fact a need, and that nursing administrators were in fact looking for something that would help them do what they had to do better. The form that the programs took also differed from program to program, but for the most part, it was a variant of the basic approach: some programs used monthly seminars, and some began to consider the feasibility of offering credit at both the undergraduate and the graduate level, as another recruitment tool and as a way of encouraging people to enter the program.

CONSTRAINTS AND STRENGTHS

At this point, it is appropriate to consider what may be called constraints and strengths. They are not really constraints, however; rather, they are things that we learned as we went through the program that must be and can be overcome before nurse administrators can be urged to move ahead. One of the things that surfaced as we began to work with people was that it takes different learners different amounts of time to complete the modules. There is an estimated timeframe put on each one of them, and the learners would find sometimes they focused on that too much. We therefore had to learn to counsel them not to be guided by that but by their own learning style, and to encourage them to be comfortable. It did take a number of them a lot of time to get through the clusters, and they tended to become discouraged. Along with that, of course, goes the faculty time that needs to be committed on a one-to-one basis to remedy the situation, which was one of the reasons we had to seek financial assistance for part-time faculty or augmented faculty time to be spent with the nurse administration. Certainly, the lack of funds to start this would seem to be a major problem, but it apparently was not, because obviously we all managed.

Available resources was something that was cited early on by the participants in the program, because the clusters within the modules do call for a lot of references. However, there were arrangements made to have all of the references made available in local VA hospitals. Moreover, all of the universities involved made sure that these references were available in their own libraries; some of them found creative ways of providing references for people who had to come long distances and were unable to get them.

Another thing that we had to learn to deal with was a variety of backgrounds. Whereas many of the nurse administrators were diploma graduates, we also had people who were master's-prepared or baccalaureate-prepared. We had to be comfortable with all of them. A problem that surfaced when they in fact came into the program and then dropped out, for whatever reason, was job pressures. In many instances that was a real problem: when they got into the program, they found that they did not have time to complete it, because they were very busy. In other instances, however, not finding time was probably a cover for being uncomfortable with the learning situations.

Another important thing that surfaced is that some of the nurse administrators cited a lack of benefit from the program. Again, this is not really a constraint; it is one of the things that we have been able to address. It became very clear that some of them were not supported by their administrators, and they were not supported by their administrators for many reasons. Some of their administrators were threatened by their becoming very knowledgeable, and some of them would not provide the dollars for them to attend the programs. We began to consider this issue in more detail as we moved into phase III.

The continuing education (CE) credit needs to be looked at; while all of the program had CE credit on it, many of these institutions would not reimburse for CE credit if they had a tuition remission program. Tuition remission in many instances was only applicable if it was in fact for credit, whether undergraduate or graduate. Consequently, many of the schools began to consider putting undergraduate or graduate credit on some of the curriculum modules, then actually did it, which helped considerably. That was a nice recruitment tool to get some of the nurse administrators into the program that they needed to go into. The universities did not standardize their charges for the different programs, however. Sometimes, participants found that if a given segment cost 500 or 600 dollars, that was a little too steep if they had to pay it out of their own pocket. As the universities worked with this, we agreed that we should begin to take a serious look at what appeared to be a lack of commitment on the part of the participants and to explore why we had so many people who would come for the self-assessment (which takes two hours and a minimum of an hour of faculty counseling) to help them decide where they needed to be and to get them oriented to a particular cluster.

We believe that the causes of these problems are things that we ultimately can do something about, and that they are outweighed by the strengths of this program. Perhaps the main strength of the program as it is presented now is that it is an adult education approach to the self-instructional curriculum that allows nurse administrators to proceed at their own pace. Once they become comfortable with the self-study design of the program, which often takes some time, it allows for a high degree of motivation and self-direction on their part. The concept of the self-assessment as a valuable learning tool cannot be too highly praised, either for individuals or for the faculty who are working with them: it helps them to identify what they need to do and then ultimately to help counsel them on where they need to go from there.

Another strength is the collaborative working relationships that have developed at multiple levels between the particular agency or facility involved and the university involved. The universities, as a result, are now known to the industry as a resource—specifically, as an educational resource—and a much stronger collaborative relationship prevails. By bringing the nursing administrators together, the universities were able to expand their own particular professional networks, which became very important to them, in that they began to realize that there were other people out there that were struggling with the same issues.

We believe that even though the program is winding down, it certainly should not be stopped. Many universities will continue to try to use these materials and continue to try to forge ahead with them. It would be a waste not to use the work that has been done and the excellent material that has been developed.

FUTURE DEVELOPMENTS

We have a few more words to say about the project. In the national survey, we found that 70 percent of nurse administrators have a diploma in nursing and that their salaries averaged about $21,000 a year. These nurses are experienced in long-term care; however, we realize that if 70 percent are graduates of hospital schools, it is possible that the level of care being given is technical. We have learned a great deal from this project; one thing we have learned is that we must begin to change the current situation, in which two thirds of nursing care is given by nursing aides, who are unlicensed, to one in which a majority of professional and associate nurses are giving skilled nursing care. Registered nurses, according to one report (U.S. Department of Health and Human Services, 1984), give about 12 minutes of nursing care a day. A good deal of their time is spent on supervision of the nursing aides.

We have years of work ahead. A few ideas about the direction of this work are pointed out by our evaluations and by the data that we are now getting about the ways and means and recommendations. Certainly, the faculty in baccalaureate and higher degree programs need to continue to work on curriculum in order to prepare their graduates to work in the field of long-term care nursing. Preparation of the faculty, nurse administrators, and professional nurses in long-term care must be addressed to a greater degree. Learning experiences also must change. Our college students are learning to be change agents. And where else should one start to help make the change but in the field of long-term care?

We need to reach out continually in our nursing organizations and universities to the long-term care agencies and organizations. We have suggested a national commission, which should be made up not only of nurses but also of long-term care representatives and consumers. A model has been set in this project for collaborative action. The universities should invite long-term care organizational representatives and nursing administrators in long-term care to sit side-by-side with faculty in their advisory committees and on their boards and plan curriculum together. We cannot make improvements in isolation: we must move into real-life situations.

Nursing organizations must become more unified and aggressive in their action. They need not only to plan for the present and the future but also to become visionaries in planning. The future is now for this kind of action. We believe that engaging consumers in the work of improvement is absolutely vital: they have considerable influence and resources. We need to get our publication units to publish the statement of roles and responsibilities and the national survey. The kind of qualifications desired for nursing personnel, as well as the nature of the nursing care to be given, should be explored in a pamphlet by professional nursing. Such a pamphlet can help the consumer of long-term care learn how to choose a nursing home. Consumers are becoming better informed and more hungry for information.

Some of the items mentioned are going to cost money, and some are not. In relation to some of them, priorities need to be changed and resources reallocated. I think that the regional associations in nursing and state nurses' associations are important in this work. They can also serve as centers for change. We have to use our resources (physical, human, and financial) more efficiently and effectively.

Planning systematically and collaboratively is essential in the years ahead. We must speak out and work energetically for change in long-term care nursing. Our elderly in this country deserve the best nursing care we can give them.

REFERENCES

Lodge, M. P. (1985). *Professional practice for nurse administrators/directors of nursing in long-term care facilities (phase I)*. Kansas City, MO: American Nurses' Foundation.

Lodge, M. P., & Pietraschke, F. (1986). *Professional education and practice of nurse administrators/directors of nursing in long-term care*. Kansas City, MO: American Nurses' Foundation.

U.S. Department of Health and Human Services, Public Health Service, Health Resources and Services Administration, Bureau of Health Professionals. (1984, May). *A report to the President and Congress on the status of health personnel in the United States*. Washington, DC: Government Printing Office.

**NURSING'S POTENTIAL
IN HEALTH CARE**

WORLDWIDE NURSING UNITY:
BUILDING A POWERHOUSE FOR CHANGE

Trevor Clay, MPhil, RGN, RMN, FRCN
General Secretary
United Kingdom's Royal College of Nursing
London, England

The advent of acquired immune deficiency syndrome (AIDS) has reminded health care providers worldwide that disease and ill health recognize no borders, that we are vulnerable, and that we must maintain constant vigilance in health all over the world. It has also stimulated some of the best international cooperation in medicine and nursing that I can remember, the lessons from which I hope we will apply in other areas.

In our different countries, we celebrate the different cultural, political, and economic systems, but I am not certain we should celebrate the difference in standards of health that exist in the world today. I believe that nursing has a duty to all of humanity regardless of borders, legal systems, and economic and political differences. However, I believe that there are danger signs in the international nursing environment at the moment.

There has always been a shortage of nurses in the developing world, and there is now a shortage in virtually all of the developed industrial nations. We have to learn from one another how we are coping with these shortages and what reforms are being undertaken. I believe that opportunities for nursing will come from our maintaining our pact with the public in our different countries and offering nursing solutions to their problems. I believe that the world nursing market should be kept as open as possible.

In the past year, we in the United Kingdom (U.K.) have seen a massive exodus of trained nurses to other countries. I have listened to British politicians suggest that our nurses ought not be allowed to go. But worse, I have listened to nurses in other countries argue that the British nurses should

Reprinted with permission from *Nursing & Health Care*. (1987). *8* (7), 407–411.

not be allowed in. I have always taken a clear view on the importance of a world that is open to nurses to take their skills wherever they are needed. To deliberately restrict the supply of nurses by closing the borders may have short-term positive effects on pay scales, but, in the long term, I think it will force the politicians and health care corporations to resort to turning to other groups for solutions to problems that urgently need solving. One of the reasons some politicians are now turning to nursing is because of the restrictive way in which the medical establishment has conducted itself.

We are at a time of change in our profession throughout the world, and the pressure of shortages will accelerate that change and make health policymakers likely to interfere in our affairs more than we might wish. To try to dilute that interference, we must be able to answer the questions the policymakers ask us, and the international environment will provide us with answers to those questions. We must all be aware of the extent to which our governments and the corporations that employ nurses work in the international environment, picking up ideas all of the time.

A COMMON AGENDA

Nursing should be a universal profession serving all of humanity, drawing inspiration from all over the world. For that to occur, it is essential that we create international links among nursing communities. I see international links as vital because, despite our many differences, I believe that we all face a common agenda for change. The starting points and the progress in different countries may vary, but that only gives us a richer selection of ideas and experiences from which to draw.

The agenda that affects us all is dominated by increasing economic and social pressures and by new ideas that press upon us all to change. We are all debating the role of nursing in health care and its relationship to the medical profession. We are all facing growing shortages of nurses. We are all debating the overwhelmingly female makeup of our profession, looking at our weaknesses and seeking new strengths. We are all engaged in arguments about the reform of nursing education. Nursing itself is examining its own leadership and development and the quality of clinical nursing practice.

OUTSIDE PRESSURES

The most powerful outside force at work on all of our health care systems is economic pressure for cost containment. As a result, in both the health care system in the United States and the socialized national health service in the U.K., cost containment has become the rule rather than the exception. Managers are beginning to challenge the judgements of the professionals, to examine the borders between the work of nurses and physicians for cost effectiveness, and to scrutinize the borders between trained nursing staff and untrained staff.

In the United States, economic pressures are leading to debates about a more socialized system of health care, about reducing the prohibitive costs of care, and about whether it is really cost effective for the society as a whole for its health service to carry a massive insurance industry on its back. We are becoming more cost conscious, but, in the U.K., we have no doubt that our National Health Service, which takes just over 6 percent of our national wealth and in return provides a service to all the people free at the point of delivery, will stand the test of economic examination. But there is a wider argument. In the U.K., it is our belief that people should have access to health care free at the point of need. In the debate over cost containment, we must assert the principles of our caring profession or be content with being selective in who we give care to.

But do the pressures from economic change amount to a revolution in health care? Looking at the international environment allows us to put matters into perspective. What has happened is that expenditures for health care in the developed world have reached a plateau, while medical advances and the graying of our population continue to make increasing demands. But even under economic constraint, the level of expenditure on health in the developed world represents untold riches to the majority of countries in the world. Our situation is difficult, but we are not necessarily in the throes of a health care revolution.

If we look at the enormity of the need for health care even in our own prosperous societies and then look at how little the boundaries between medicine and nursing have moved, it is possible to argue that we have only made marginal changes. We have not addressed the great priorities and choices in health care delivery. We talk about priorities, about the importance of primary health care, about promotion and prevention, but our systems remain overwhelmingly dominated by the institutional secondary health care model, and the vast majority of nurses work inside those institutions running a sickness service rather than a health service.

I am not arguing for a romantic return to the community by the vast army of nurses who work in hospitals. One lesson we have learned from the success in tackling the great epidemics such as smallpox and cholera and in ensuring that our children get through childhood healthy and through most of their lives without pain is that they still face the likelihood of ill health before they die. We have eradicated tuberculosis; people now die of heart disease, cancer, and strokes, or they have their independence taken away by Alzheimer's disease, which cripples the mind but leaves the body to be nursed. The majority of nurses in our systems will continue to work in hospitals, and we must ensure that we prepare them adequately for the task.

We also face outside pressures on health care from population changes. I do not want to dwell on the graying of the population, but in the U.K., the average 30-year-old only costs our health service \$250 per year. An average person over 65 costs the service \$2,270 per year. There is no cure for old age, and the demand for nursing services will continue to rise in all our countries to the turn of the century.

The other end of the population equation that is causing nursing a problem throughout the developed world is the drop in the number of young women graduating from college and the competition for their employment from other professions. Women have different needs from the health services. They are often the most vocal segments of a consumer movement that is questioning and challenging the profession.

Economic changes, population changes, and changes in social attitudes have changed the environments in which we all work. We have tried different ways to cope with the changes with varying degrees of success. There is much that we can learn from one another.

INTERNAL PRESSURES

The outside pressures on the provision of health care and the practice of nursing are great, but the pressures inside nursing are no less strong.

In every country I have visited, the role of nursing is being debated. Health care priorities are shifting away from major institutions and the treatment of sick individuals and towards primary health care and ensuring that key groups such as elderly persons and mentally handicapped persons receive as much care as is possible in the community.

The World Health Organization has acknowledged that nursing will play the leading role in primary health care. So as the philosophies of care change, policymakers reassess the role of nursing. Within limited budgets, those policymakers and legislators are being forced to recognize that nursing combines the necessary level of skill for the job with affordability.

But with change comes resistance, especially from some of our medical colleagues and sometimes from within our own profession. I believe that the best health care is given when teamwork between medicine and nursing and all the other contributors is seen as cooperation among equals.

When nurses consider extended roles in either hospitals or in communities, we must take a realistic view of the limits of our competence. But a realistic view of nursing competence that draws on the international environment provides a host of examples: the independent roles of Britain's health visitors, home nursing service, and midwifery service: the public health nurses in Finland; the many extended roles that have evolved as much through necessity as planning in the Third World; and America's nurse practitioners give us a huge body of knowledge from which to draw in arguments about the future.

Ironically, the successes of the medical profession are the greatest threat to its dominance in health care delivery. As medical research provides new drugs, new procedures, and new tests, the practitioners go on to simplify and modify them. As it becomes better established, a new treatment, process, or drug requires less and less medical training to make it work and, invariably, nursing staff members begin to administer it. These developments are unstoppable and in due course nurses' time will come and our competence will be recognized. I have learned a great deal from American nurses' struggles with the medical profession, where cooperation has been tried and failed and nursing is now seeking legislative change. Nurses in the U. K. are just beginning to go down that road and may soon have our first legislation on nurse prescribing.

NURSING LEADERSHIP

In our different organizations, the debate about where the leadership in nursing really lies is heating up. Nursing throughout the world is a hierarchical profession with tremendous tensions within it among the clinical nurses, who provide the backbone of continuing service in a wide range of settings; the new and emerging specialists, who often have their own narrow areas of concern; the educators, who argue for change to be preceded by reform in nursing education; and, finally, the managers of nursing, with their day-to-day control of the service and their preoccupation with staffing and hospitals and delivering a service.

Nurse managers in the U.K. are increasingly being overruled by general managers and budget holders. Their ability to lead the profession is seriously under challenge from both within and outside of nursing. They stand accused by other nurses of being prepared in many cases to dilute the skill mix by using untrained staff members or student nurses. They also stand accused of being out of touch with practice. The managers feel they are the defenders of the profession against the pressures of the real world.

The educators in the U.K., who for the past twenty years have been preparing to move nursing education into more mainstream education and away from the use and abuse of students in the service, stand accused of elitism and denying the realities of caring for patients. Physicians in the U.K. return from the United States with dark stories of the terrible things that happen when they work with American nurses with baccalaureate and higher degrees. Apparently the physicians find that those American nurses talk back.

The nursing specialists have given much to the profession and have taken the levels of our work up to new heights, but other nurses accuse them of shaping their practices to the parameters of medical specialties and working as high-level support workers to medicine rather than providing a nursing service to patients. There is evidence that physicians see the specialists' roles this way as well. When new budgeting experiments were being carried out in the U.K., a physician on one pilot project in an intensive therapy unit (ITU) was in favor of reducing the number of ITU nurses and replacing them with less-expensive technicians.

While the managers, the educators, and the specialists argue about the future of the profession, many of the practitioners are demonstrating in practice the wider roles that nurses can perform. Many of these roles go beyond the competencies laid out by the managers and the educators. Studies in Australia and in the U.K. have consistently shown that, in practice, physicians and nurses are developing new departures in care and treatment whether the hierarchies of their professions approve or not.

So where does the leadership in nursing lie? It is my experience in the U. K. that it does not lie with any group in the profession, but instead with individuals whose experience bridges more than one of the groups, or in one of the organizations whose membership unites the forces in nursing that have so often worked against one another in the past.

I believe that the new circumstances we face in our countries demand that we produce a new breed of leaders in nursing and that we tackle the hierarchy and divisions in our professions. We must also work to keep new divisions from emerging.

I believe that this must come through changes in the clinical setting and in the education of future generations of nurses. Their education must unite work in the community with work in hospitals, and it must give nurses a sound understanding of all of the major branches of nursing. But if we educate the new breed of nurse, it will be for nothing if they are then thrown into clinical settings where there are the old divisions between clinical nurses and educators, where managers keep their hands off patients, and where specialists keep to themselves and cross fertilization is absent. Too often, nurses perceive leadership as providing a victory for one part of nursing over another. True leadership looks at the demands for health care and then brings all the parts of nursing together to present a solution—our solution—to the policymakers.

What I think we need is a broader education for our nurses, followed by experience of a flatter structure in health care delivery by giving flexibility in nursing and greater integration and cross fertilization among ourselves than we have enjoyed up until now.

PRESSURES CAUSE DIVISIVENESS

I believe that for all of us to face the agenda we have in common internationally, we must face it with unity. However, as I have said, with change comes resistance, and the resistance to progress in nursing is great. I see four main pressures that divide the family of nursing—they are politics, labor relations, client groups, and specializations.

In many countries, political divisions obstruct the work of nursing, especially where, as we have in the U.K., some nursing organizations attach themselves to a political party and expect the fortunes of nursing to rise and fall with the political tide. That is a form of political involvement that I do not think takes us very far forward.

I strongly support political involvement, and I think there is much we can learn from one another about the ways in which we influence our different governments. I am impressed with the pressure that nursing organizations in the United States are able to bring to bear on the legislators. As a profession, we must be much more outward looking now that outside forces and politcal progress decide so much that happens in health care. I think it is essential that nurses understand how they can get involved in political life and why it is essential for our profession's future.

Looking at nursing organizations throughout the world, the nursing profession is divided over its labor relations leadership. Some nurses belong to general unions, joining in common cause with other health care workers; others belong to nurse-only organizations. Many nurses belong to what they see as professional organizations that do not involve themselves in pay bargaining. The division between professional and trade union work I see throughout the world disturbs me. Being a profession is about controlling all aspects of that profession. It is an illusion to imagine that levels of pay do not have a crucial impact on the success or failure of important developments in nursing as a whole.

Unity of activities is essential to change. We must deal with the need of both the practice of nursing and the practitioner. We understand that they are different, but we should not delude ourselves that progress can be made without the needs of both nurses and nursing being debated and resolved together.

I am disturbed by what I see as division in nursing based on broad client groups or settings. I believe that hospital- and community-based nurses still have more in common than they have differences to divide them. In the U.K.-approach to reforming nursing education, we have not gone down the road of the "generic nurse," but we have sought to ensure that the common training of nurses is broadly based enough to give students contact with all branches of nursing.

I understand fully the organizational and practical difficulties there are in creating both professional and trade union unity within a single organization, but I am concerned that some of those divisions are now beginning to spill onto the international scene. All I bring you is our experience from the U.K., where I think we have come closer than anywhere else to resolving the dilemma of combining all of these parts of the profession's activities into one organization.

U.K. APPROACH

We have all of the internal nursing arguments in the U.K. that nurses in America have. The difference is we have them within one organization, and we have mechanisms for resolving them. We do not leave ourselves open to be divided and ruled by politicians and other professions when we tackle a major policy issue in health. We find that the tension we get is creative, not destructive. There is nothing more destructive than disunity.

There is one particular reason that I believe that maximum unity is important. The vast majority of the members of nursing organizations throughout the world are women. Despite our best efforts, the profession of nursing is still seen in most countries as being of a low status. Our members suffer from all the obstacles to full participation in political and professional life that the women's movement has highlighted over the past 20 years. Many women already have their lives divided between work and home, carrying the burden of two jobs. If we add to that a further set of divisions in the organizations they must join if they are to express themselves politically, then we will disadvantage them even further. We will restrict full participation in nursing to a mobile, often single, well-paid few. We also then risk the fact that many nurses will give priority to only one aspect of nursing—their pay negotiations. In so many of the changes we want to bring about, we need all of the members of our huge profession that we can get behind us.

STRENGTHENING THE LINKS

I would like to close by offering some proposals about ways in which we can strengthen nursing's international links.

First, as I have said, I want to see more international mobility among nurses. In particular, I would like to see more opportunities for student nurses to travel as part of their educations. In some parts of Europe, this is done with much success. I think it is greatly to the credit of the United States that when American nurses partake in educational events at home or abroad, they are given educational credit for it. Our system in the U.K. has not yet awakened to this important incentive to travel and learn.

Second, I want to see barriers to nurses working in different countries kept to a minimum. Countries should not hide behind false arguments about standards and quality. Various extra qualifications are excellent in themselves, but it is a weak argument that says that nurses cannot practice in particular countries because especially high standards are needed. If that was the case, there would be no nurses in Beirut, where the demands being made on nursing standards exceed our wildest nightmares. Where the doors are open, nurses will always rise to the challenges beyond them.

Third, I would like to see much more comparative research in which the researchers look in real depth at whether innovations in one country are appropriate for another. At the moment in the U.K., we are trying to reform nursing education. There is a barrage of ill-informed comment about what happened in Australia when they reformed the system in one of their states, but little that is authoritative.

I congratulate nursing in the United States on ushering in a National Center for Nursing Research within the National Institutes of Health, and on defending the federal funding for it. It seems obvious to me that we need more international research exchange, where research could be coordinated over several countries and the results compared. The nursing profession of the world is large enough to merit this sort of effort.

Fourth, I would like to see communications through the popular nursing journals improved dramatically. We live in a global village, but reporting of international nursing issues remains very weak.

Finally, I would like to see a focus on the developing world. As our philosophies of care change, many of you will feel, as I do, the burden of our history and the institutions and patterns of care we have inherited holding back change. How often have we wished that we could start from a different point? Many of our colleagues in the developing world, however, are closer to that position. I believe that they also face many of the basic questions about priorities for care. We need a clear international mechanism for keeping in touch with developments in their countries, for I think that the flow of ideas will be from them to us and that we have the most to learn. I believe that we have that mechanism in the ICN, and we must build upon it with urgency not only to exchange ideas, but to support one another in as many ways as possible.

Dr. Mahler, the director of the World Health Organization, has said of nurses and primary health care, "If millions of nurses in a thousand different places articulate the same ideas and convictions about primary health care and come together as one force, they could act as a powerhouse for change." I believe that, together, we are that powerhouse for change.

AN UPDATE ON THE NATIONAL COMMISSION ON NURSING IMPLEMENTATION PROJECT: NURSING OPPORTUNITIES

Vivien DeBack, PhD, RN
Project Director
National Commission on Nursing Implementation Project
Milwaukee

In this paper, I will briefly discuss some ideas on nursing's potential in the health care industry that have been brought together by staff and workgroup members of the National Commission on Nursing Implementation Project (NCNIP). This project, directed by organized nursing, is responsible for implementing key recommendations from two major studies completed in 1983, namely, the reports on nursing of the National Commission on Nursing and the Institute of Medicine. Among the three goals of the NCNIP is the identification and continued development of high-quality, cost-effective nurse-managed systems. To accomplish this goal, the NCNIP has over the past two years

- Collected data on present nursing delivery systems;
- Reviewed documents compiled by futurists based on present trends to determine the types of systems needed for the future;
- Identified the differences between the future and now; and
- Discovered, by the case-study method, systems that demonstrate factors that are considered to be necessary for the high-quality, cost-effective nurse-managed systems of the future.

Through a number of site visits and self-reports by project workgroup members, a considerable amount of anecdotal data has been collected. In what follows, I offer some of what has been learned by staff and workgroup members of this project for the purpose of increasing our common understanding of nursing systems of the future and opportunities for nurses in those systems.

HISTORY

In the past, nursing's activities have been identified by the sites in which nurses worked. Nurses who worked in hospitals, nursing homes, schools, and offices performed certain duties that were considered to be necessary in those environments. As a result, the systems determined what nurses did; neither nurses themselves or the profession as a whole determined what nurses could do. There are several reasons why this was so.

1. Nurses have not described their practice differences. That is, institutions and agencies who hire nurses are not clear as to the differences in practice between nurses, physicians, social workers, and other therapists.
2. Nurses have not identified costs for their services, and thus appropriate pricing of those services cannot be done. Furthermore, the lack of cost data on nursing services leaves nursing in a position of being unable to prove cost-effectiveness.
3. Nursing has not identified outcomes of patient care that are the result of nursing intervention. Therefore, organizations that hire nurses are not aware of the benefits of nursing care to their agency mission.

The health care system will continue to determine what nurses do unless nurses describe their practice, identifying what the client and organization receives from nurses and what those services cost.

A TABLE OF SYSTEMS IN WHICH NURSES WORK

Based on information from the NCNIP, a beginning description of the systems in which nurses work has been developed. The table of systems provides a new framework for looking at arenas of care and addresses nursing's role in each of those arenas (see Table 1). As presently identified, there are three care types of models of care: (1) medical, (2) interdisciplinary, and (3) nursing. None of these models is better than either of the others: they are simply different. Because they are different, they make different demands on practitioners.

THE MEDICAL MODEL

In the medical model, the physician is the predominant director of care, and the focus of the service is cure or treatment of acute illness. The system has the mission of cure with a medical orientation. Therefore, nurses become quite frustrated when they try to overlay a nursing model on a medical system. What is needed here is for nurses to identify themselves as collaborators in a system whose goal is a medical outcome. Here is a critical setting in which nurses can define what they do that is different from what physicians do—specifically, what it is that they contribute to the organizational outcome, and what the cost of services provided by nurses will be.

Table 1 describes types of settings in which we may expect to see a medical model of care. It is not an exhaustive list, and it does not imply that all agencies of this type follow medical models of care. It is important to note that it is not the site that determines the model but rather the professional that is responsible for making the care decisions—in the case of the medical model, the physician.

THE INTERDISCIPLINARY MODEL

In the interdisciplinary model, the team directs the care. The team can be any combination of health care professionals, including nurses, social workers, physicians, occupational therapists, and the like. The focus of care is rehabilitation or "community" care. In this system the client's needs drive the decision-making process. The professional with the expertise to respond to the clients needs becomes the major care provider, but the decisions are team-determined. Each professional brings his or her experience and background to the team and can become a major player in care planning. The team as a whole plans and evaluates the care. Nurses and nursing care are part of the team and team activities.

There are a number of advantages for nursing in the interdisciplinary model of care. Nursing is incorporated into all aspects of care and decision making. Nurses may be the major care providers, and they are collegial with all other providers. It is true that collegiality is frequently found in a medical model of care; however, such models are not interdisciplinary, because the decision-making power remains with the physician.

There are also disadvantages to the interdisciplinary model. Nursing may lose its uniqueness, because care is provided by all professionals on the team, including nurses. In some interdisciplinary models, a case management system is in place, and the nurses are the case managers. In these systems the uniqueness of nursing is not lost.

Table 1 describes a number of settings in which interdisciplinary models of care may be found. Again, this is not an exhaustive list, nor does it describe all agencies of this type.

NURSING MODEL

In the nursing model, the director of care and decision maker is the nurse. The foci of care are health promotion, health maintenance, and illness prevention. In this system, the nurses identify very clearly what they do, what the client can expect from them, and what it costs, because nursing is the system. Obviously, theoretical nursing models fit very well into this system. Nurses, along with clients, identify health care needs. Plans for meeting those needs are formulated, and nurses then provide the services or obtain services from other providers for the client.

The types of settings listed in Table 1 are some of the arenas in which the nursing model of care may be operational.

CONCLUSION

The system or model of care in any health care setting will determine where resources will be spent. Nurses who are aware of the sytem in which they work will be more effective in complementing the system with the expertise they can provide. Nurses may find that attempting to identify health promotion as a major focus in a hospital setting where the focus of care is cure of an illness may meet with resistance. Comments of "We can't afford that" or "There is not enough staff" can be expected. However, if we match the service with the focus of care, or broaden the focus of care, the response may be different. All of the models identified in Table 1 are driven by the purposes of the organization or agency and of whoever they determine are their clients. There needs to be a fit between the mission of the institution, the goals of the group, and the client needs.

Whatever the system, the point of analyzing their component parts is to optimize the role of nurses within the system. Unless nurses understand and lead the system (relative to nursing care), they will be led by it.

ACKNOWLEDGMENTS

Thanks are expressed to Margaret Murphy, MS, RN, Staff Specialist, National Commission on Nursing Implementation Project, for the ideas and the table of systems presented in this paper.

Table 1. Systems in Which Nurses Work

Care Model	Predominant Director of Care	Focus of Care	Types of Settings
Medical	MD	Cure/treat illness	Hospital HMO Independent/ group practice Surgical/ emergency centers
Inter-disciplinary	Team (SW, NSE, MD, OT, etc.)	Rehabilitation, "community" care	Rehabilitation institution Public Health Joint practice Psychiatric hospital
Nursing	Nurse	Health promotion Health maintenance Illness prevention	Home care Nursing home Nusing clinic Visiting nurse association Independent practice Birthing centers

ASSOCIATE DEGREE NURSING AND HEALTH CARE

Margaret H. Applegate, EdD, RN
Associate Dean for Associate Degree Programs
Indiana University School of Nursing
Indianapolis

The purpose of this paper is to review the history of associate degree nursing, paying attention to the current state of affairs and the vital link between associate degree nursing and health care in the future. In reviewing literature with this in mind, it became apparent that we are at last on the threshold of the nursing future that Dr. Mildred Montag envisioned in 1952. Nursing is just beginning to emerge as a science. Its history is as a technology rooted in the medical model (Swenson, 1972). Montag transformed that model into a nursing model and provided the foundation for differentiated practice that can both liberate the professional nurse and secure the future of the technical nurse toward the goal of enhanced health care in a changing environment. We need but review the origins of associate degree nursing and its progress to be conscious of its current importance to the future of health care.

HISTORICAL BACKGROUND

In the early 1900s and through the first half of the 20th century, the nursing education model was dominated by hospital-based diploma programs. In 1949, nearly 87 percent of nursing education programs were based in hospital schools, and only 13 percent in collegiate schools (Swenson, 1972). The model of education was largely apprenticeship training that provided both service to the hospital and training for students. Since the students' experience was dictated by service needs, it was largely unplanned (Rines, 1977). Programs improved in quality over the years, though the curricula continued to reflect the medical model and hospital geography. Diploma programs produced the majority of nurses, who served the profession well, and prepared individuals who rose through personal talent to the leadership ranks of nursing. A changing health care system, economics, and the drive to move nursing into institutions of higher education suggest that it is time to move to a new era in nursing education. Indeed, the movement is under way.

Events around World War II marked a period of major change in the nursing world. There was a serious shortage of nurses to meet the needs of the home front and the war effort. Congress passed legislation, the Bolton Act, to create a Student War Nursing Reserve, which came to be called the Cadet Nurse Corps (Rines, 1977). Nursing programs accelerated, and class enrollments increased. At that time, Montag developed a Cadet Corps program at Adelphi College in which she introduced many of the characteristics that would later define associate degree nursing. This experience made it clear that qualified nurses could be prepared in less than three years.

Many studies of nursing were done after World War II. Brown (1948) surveyed nursing schools in this country and recommended, among other things, that nursing education move into the mainstream of the educational system. Many similar reports supported her recommendations. At the same time, Canada was experimenting with nursing education models to determine whether or not professional nurses could be prepared in two years (Rines, 1977).

During this same period, community colleges began to proliferate to meet the needs of servicemen and servicewomen returning to civilian life, as well as the personnel needs stimulated by technological advances (Perkins, 1983). These institutions provided instruction in the sciences and humanities for students who were enrolled in local diploma programs. In 1949, the American Association of Junior Colleges and the National League for Nursing Education began to study the role of community colleges in nursing education. These two organizations would ultimately form a joint committee that continued until 1986.

Within this context, Montag published a book in 1951, based on her doctoral studies, that assessed the existing nursing education system and its implications for vocational and technical nursing education (Rines, 1977). She was concerned about the adequacy of the preparation of practical nurses to meet emerging health care needs. At the same time, she was convinced that through controlled education registered nurses could be prepared more effectively in a shorter period of time than the three years required for hospital-based programs. Thus the idea was born.

In 1952 the Cooperative Research Project in Junior and Community College Education for Nursing was funded by an anonymous donor, and the associate degree in nursing (ADN) program was initiated under Montag's leadership. The purpose of the project was to develop and test a new type of program to prepare men and women for those functions commonly associated with the registered nurse (Montag, 1959). At its inception, Montag envisioned two types of nurses, professional and technical, with a third assisting category. She has since stated that the development of the professional programs should have occurred at the same time, to allow both programs to emerge simultaneously with clearly differentiated functions (Montag, 1980). Had that occurred, nursing might have had a different history. The basic assumptions for the project were as follows.

- "The functions of nursing can and should be differentiated into three basic categories: the professional, the semiprofessional or technical, and the assisting.
- The great bulk of nursing functions lie in the intermediate category, the semiprofessional or technical.
- Education for nursing belongs within the organized educational framework.
- When preparation for nursing is education rather than service-centered, the time required may be reduced." (Montag, 1959)

The project was a curriculum study organized as action research, in which the faculty of the participating programs developed autonomous curricula within guiding principles and parameters, and the project staff served as consultants. It was national in scope and resulted in the only type of nursing education to arise from planned research and experimentation (Rines, 1977).

After the project, in 1957, the National League for Nursing hired a series of educators to assist community colleges in developing ADN programs with the aid of Sealantic funds. In 1959 further funding was made available through the Kellogg Foundation four-state project to expand and enhance associate degree programs and to prepare faculty to teach in them. Careful planning, excellent funding, and a ready social climiate provided a base for the rapid proliferation of these programs. In 1952 there were two, in 1969 there were over 400, and by 1985 there were 777 ADN programs in this country. Bullough (1979) noted that associate degree graduates constitute a major portion of the nursing workforce. Associate degree education has emerged as the predominant model for the education of the basic registered nurse.

Several attributes of the pilot programs came to characterize associate degree nursing and to change the face of nursing education in this nation (Montag, 1959; Anderson, 1966; Rines, 1977).

- The programs were integral components of colleges.
- The focus of nursing care changed to a nursing model dealing with nursing responses to patient problems using a broad fields approach.
- Faculty were hired, promoted, and evaluated according to the same criteria as other faculty in the college.
- Nontraditional students with a heterogeneous learner profile were drawn to nursing and admitted according to the same criteria as other students in the college.

- General education was integrated into the curriculum to enhance individual growth as well as occupational readiness.

- Learning was controlled and goal-directed and employed innovative teaching strategies.

The ADN programs and products were among the most studied and evaluated in history. Competencies were developed carefully to define the product. The curriculum was delivered as a total package, not just a collection of courses. Sequence became important rather than random enrollment.

COMPETENCIES AND SCOPE OF PRACTICE

Competencies of associate degree nurses have been defined, redefined, and tested repeatedly over the years. One of the finest contributions of associate degree education to nursing is its clear delineation of the role of the technical nurse. It has forced the profession to study and define the professional role (Rines, 1977). This has contributed to the acceptance of the need for the professional to reach beyond the technical role and take the actions necessary to seek sanction for that expanded role. That sanction has been difficult to achieve, especially in structured settings.

Recently the National Commission on Nursing Implementation Project (NCNIP) studied associate degree and baccalaureate competency statements developed by various funded and unfunded projects (DeBack, 1986). The purpose was to analyze a sample of national, regional, and state-derived statements to identify areas of consensus and nonconsensus regarding common and differentiating competencies. Although the sample did not constitute the universe of competencies, it was broad enough to discern a growing consensus regarding them. The major differences noted between ADN and bachelor of science in nursing (BSN) products were related to the type of client served (patient condition) and the environment for practice (structure and support). These were consistent with the commonly held ADN competencies, as were the majority of those considered to be common to both groups. Areas still open to debate include such things as the ADN role in nursing diagnosis, patient teaching, evaluation of care, and delegation.

The nursing diagnosis debate centers on who is to derive the diagnosis, the use of standardized nursing diagnoses, distinctions between nursing diagnoses and clinical problems, and the need for technical nurses to be skilled in rendering nursing diagnoses relevant to the individual patient. Teaching issues follow the same general format. There seems to be a consensus that the professional nurse is responsible for long-range teaching plans and standardized teaching plans. Who should assume responsibility for short-term teaching plans and individualization of plans is still under debate, though most associate degree advocates would consider this area to be appropriate to the technical role. A serious concern is when and where teaching will occur.

The acuity level of the patients in acute care-settings clearly affects the determination of the teachable moment. As the health care system is increasingly driven by a protocol-based delivery model, these issues may be resolved with less difficulty.

Management and leadership is also an unclear area. There is a consensus that the leadership role rests with the professional nurse, though it is unclear what level of preparation of the professional nurse is appropriate to this role. The questions arise in the discussion of patient care management and delegation functions. Varying definitions of patient care management cloud the issue further.

Much of the work on role differentiation has been done on the basis of current practice and the present view of health care, rather than of a futures perspective to guide nursing practice needs and goals. Through the collaborative efforts of members of the major nursing organizations, consumers, and representatives of groups that influence nursing, the National Commission on Nursing has reviewed the literature and conducted debates to develop descriptions of the professional and technical nurse of the future. The intent was not to decrease the technical role but to expand the professional role to meet the health care needs of society in the future (NCNIP, 1987).

A consensus on competencies is emerging, and it is critical to the current issues before us. It is the responsibility of the professional organizations to define scope of practice, but that scope will be influenced significantly by competency statements. Both the NLN and the ANA have developed competency statements. The ANA and various states are struggling with scope of practice statements. Currently the major organizations are collaborating on scope of practice statements to seek a consensus. Clearly, it is emerging; just as clearly, it is not yet settled. It is crucial that scope of practice statements be sufficiently broad to provide for the dynamic state of nursing while providing the clarity needed to differentiate.

The movement from competencies to scope of practice and then to licensure and titling issues has been painfully slow. One reason is that the competencies have been used more to guide education than to guide practice. The work world has continued to operate largely in the technical sphere and has failed to use vocational, technical, or professional nurses differently, to a large extent. This continues to blur roles and foster discontent. Few nurses are afforded the satisfaction of the efficient and effective use of the differentiated roles in a complementary manner. The current need is for demonstration studies of differentiated practice. Until this occurs, the issue cannot be resolved.

Several studies recently have been concluded or are underway to test competencies in practice. Waters and Limon (1987) completed a three-year project in California designed to validate the NLN statements as accurate descriptors of ADN competencies. Six demonstration sites were used to implement miniprojects to test the validity of the descriptors in specific roles or, in some cases, all five roles identified in the NLN statements. Although some variation was found in individual projects, overall findings supported the contention that the NLN competency statements describe entry-level performance behaviors of ADN graduates.

Rotkovitch (1986) and colleagues are conducting a study to test whether the educational preparation of ADN and BSN graduates, as reflected by expected behaviors, can be integrated into practice. They call their model ICON (integrated competencies of nursing). They are testing the use of three member teams, each comprising two ADN-prepared nurses and one BSN-prepared nurse, to deliver care in acute-care settings. The size and composition of teams would be expected to vary according to the setting and the patient profile. They have both a transitional model and a futures model in place on two test units. In the transitional model, experienced ADN, diploma, and BSN graduates practice under the professional job description, and newly graduated ADN, BSN, and diploma graduates function under an associate nurse job description. After a minimum orientation of six months, BSN graduates become eligible to practice under the professional job description. Practical nurses who are assessed as being exceptionally strong are given additional inservice education preparation in pharmacology, nursing process, and selected skills, and are then permitted to practice under the associate nurse job description. This approach will be interesting to watch, because it has implications for grandfathering. Further studies will have to reach beyond exceptional practical nurses if conclusions are to be generalized.

On the futures unit, only ADN and BSN nurses are employed in the differentiated roles. The BSN nurse is responsible for coordination of the care of the patients assigned to the team, for the overall plan of care, and for the delegation of care to the ADN nurse. The ADN nurse is the main caregiver and is responsible for assessing the patients' response to care and for collaborating with the BSN nurse in evaluating patient care outcomes and mofifying the plan of care accordingly. The associate degree nurse is expected to interact directly with all members of the health team, participate in discharge planning, and teach patients and families within the framework of an established teaching plan, among other competencies listed. No delegation role is listed. The project will measure quality of care delivered, cost-effectiveness, staffing effectiveness, and job satisfaction in differentiated roles. This study is in its early stages, and outcomes are just beginning to emerge. Any conclusions, therefore, would be premature.

Primm (1986) was the project director for the MAIN/Kellogg projects: "Facilitating ADN Competency Development" and "Defining and Differentiating ADN and BSN Competency Development." These competencies currently are being tested in the service setting through use of differentiated job descriptions. These job descriptions identify competencies in three major areas: direct client care, communication, and management of care. Primm suggests that until service differentiates between the two categories of practice, the reality gap will continue.

ROLE DIFFERENTIATION

Why two categories of nursing? The role of the nurse is already too broad, and it continues to grow in both breadth and complexity in an environment of radical change. The functions of the nurse are too many and various to be embraceable by a single worker. Montag (1980) envisioned the functions of nursing along a continuum, with professional nursing at one end and assisting personnel at the other. The technical nurse was defined through functions in the midrange of the continuum. Although commonalities of function occur, the role of the professional was seen as being greater in depth and scope and as both embracing and reaching beyond the common core of practice.

The need for and effectiveness of the ADN nurse has been well established and documented. The ADN nurse was proposed and developed as a new worker prepared to fulfill the technical nursing functions (Anderson, 1966). It is critical that we learn to use that nurse in the manner in which he or she was prepared, so that the full value of the role can be appreciated. Brown (1948) cautioned against understanding the ability of the technician in either knowledge or practice. Waters (1965) noted that there are compelling reasons for making distinctions between technical and professional performance: our students, our patients, our employers, and ourselves. She further notes that the persistence of both ADN and BSN programs and the market demand for the products imply a belief that there is a difference in the products and that both are desirable.

It is difficult to understand why differentiated practice has been so slow in evolving. Certainly the shortage of nurses has played a significant role. Until the supply of nurses is sufficient in the desired mix, differentiated practice will be difficult. As associate degree nurses moved into the health care arena, there were few professional nurses prepared at the baccalaureate level to serve as models of professional nursing and few service sanctions to reinforce such practice. This too discouraged differentiated practice. The failure to define the professional nurse at that time and the tendency to group the associate and diploma nurses together caused further delays (Huber, 1982).

As ADN nurses were stretched through assignment beyond their preparation, faculties began to expand the curriculum to meet the reality of the work world and the demands of service. Some evolving changes, such as inclusion of patient teaching and conversion of the problem-solving process to a structured nursing process, were useful and consistent with a changing environment. The addition of community health and leadership often required extension of the time needed for the program, or a compromise of some of the basic knowledge and skill components of the program accompanied by an erosion of the original philosophy of technical nursing education. Electives or postgraduation preparation for extended expectations in particular geographic regions might have been a more useful way of responding to the needs of the local community without changing the preservice education program in such a dramatic way. Indeed, some programs used this approach. Failure to utilize the available professional nurses effectively in such areas as coordination and case management, policy-making and protocol development, and long-range planning have led to dissatisfaction and increased confusion and role diffusion.

Until we differentiate clearly between graduates and use them in practice accordingly, the two categoreis of nurses will continue to be adversaries. Only through proper utilization will mutual respect, complementary roles, and collaborative care emerge. As Voltaire once said, "A long dispute means both parties are wrong." We have disputed too long.

TITLING AND LICENSURE

Titling and licensure continues to be an area of dispute. At this point in our history, we must be ready to unite and resolve this issue. The greatest contribution technical nursing can make to the discipline is the liberation of the professional nurse. Associate degree nurses have a strong and successful record in the midrange of nursing functions: they have demonstrated consistent success on the NCLEX-RN, which measures technical competence. The ADN scope of practice and demonstration of safe practice measured by the NCLEX-RN licensure exam must continue if professional nursing is to be freed to address the ever-expanding continuum that represents the universe of nursing practice.

The professional nurse must be licensed through a separate and distinct examination that measures the total scope of professional nursing practice. The professional practitioner must be free to expand nursing knowledge and to provide leadership in nursing education, practice, and research. In the absence of a competent technical nurse, that will not be possible.

How to achieve unity on licensure is a knotty problem. Licensure is, of course, a state's right, and the issue certainly will be fought out in that arena. Without a national guiding force, this could lead to chaos and seriously hamper the geographic mobility of nurses. The ANA and the NLN have been involved in the licensure issue from the very beginning. As a result of the efforts of the organizations that would evolve into the ANA and the NLN in cooperation with the International Congress of Nurses and Ethel Fenwich, the first licensure statute for nursing became a reality in 1903 in North Carolina (Fondiller, 1986). As we struggle with this issue today, the nursing organizations can, through position statements and resolutions, continue to provide the leadership that will guide states to a unified position. We are those organizations. Through our membership, our voice, and our vote, we can control our own destiny.

The NLN proposed the NCLEX-RN licensure for associate degree nurses and a separate and distinct license for the professional nurse at its 1987 convention. This proposal would enable scope of practice to be maintained in a manner consistent with that measurement of safe practice, and the titling issue might become less difficult.

An issue of great concern that remains unresolved is that of grandfathering or waivering. A grandfather clause is a statutory or regulatory provision to exempt from newly imposed requirements those individuals already engaged in the field who may be presumed to possess the necessary qualifications. It is used to protect the property rights of the individual vis-a-vis his or her licensure. A waiver clause, on the other hand, is a statutory or regulatory provision whereby some or all requirements for licensure are lifted in some cases for a fixed period of time. If there is a waiver of new requirements, equivalency criteria must be provided (NCSBN, 1986).

Grandfathering, waivering, or grandfathering with waiver clauses will be established on a state-by-state basis. This issue could also create serious endorsement problems as nurses attempt to move from state to state. Some states could require that endorsement applicants meet the same requirements as applicants for initial licensure. Others might require an endorsement applicant to meet the requirements in the endorsing state at the time of the applicant's original licensure (NCSBN, 1986). Equivalency criteria could vary from state to state. These issues will require careful consideration. Nurses must begin now to study grandfathering and waiver mechanisms so that they can communicate knowledgably as the debate ensues. Regional workshops on this issue would surely capture a wide audience.

There seems to be a general consensus that ADN, diploma, and BSN graduates should be grandfathered into the professional role. Indeed, the RN license that they hold is a constitutional right guaranteed under the 14th amendment, and it would not be disturbed. However, a new and distinct license for the professional would raise new questions around this issue.

The controversy primarily has to do with licensed practical nurses and whether they should be grandfathered into the role of the technical nurse of the future. There are strong views on both sides of this issue. Several scenarios have been proposed for consideration, and more are sure to emerge. Proponents of one view would grandfather (or waiver) all practical nurses into the new technical role. This view assumes that nursing service administrators, or some other designated body, would either upgrade the preparation of practical nurses or keep sufficient records to use them differently. Clearly, equivalency criteria would be needed, as well as extensive monitoring mechanisms. Methods and costs of assessment and necessary education could prove to be problematic in this model. If all practical nurses were to be grandfathered, 63 percent of all technical nurses would have received no education beyond the LPN level by the year 2000 (ANA, 1987).

Another option would allow current practical nurses to take the examination for licensure to practice as a technical nurse. Those who passed the examination would be employed to function within that scope of practice; those who did not would either continue to practice as practical nurses in positions requiring that scope of practice or would be free to enter mobility programs to prepare to take the technical or the professional examination, depending on the program selected for further education. A transition timeline would be necessary in this model. It is assumed to affect the current practical nurse population; it does not imply the continuation of LPN programs.

Still another scenario would not prepare additional practical nurses, but would not grandfather those in practice or allow them to take the technical nurse examination without additional educational preparation. It would encourage flexible mobility options that recognize past learning and experience for those who would wish to advance to a new role. This option and the one just before it assume that there will be a continuing role for a declining number of practical nurses in the near future.

Other options are sure to exist, and each will have both advantages and disadvantages. The legal implications of grandfathering have not yet been explored fully. At this point in nursing's history, there is little case law to guide either deliberations or decision making on this issue. Regardless of the positions taken or conclusions reached, this issue will continue to be a difficult one.

PRESENT AND FUTURE CHANGE

Change will come as surely as it has over the centuries. As Margaret Mead (1963) has said, "No one will live all his life in the world into which he was born, and no one will die in the world in which he worked in his maturity." We are all aware of the changes in the health care system, with prospective payment, emerging systems for outpatient and home care, a corporate and competitive health system model, expanding technology, an aging society, increased patient acuity in acute-care settings, a rapid increase in extended care facilities, growing ethical dilemmas, and a myriad of other issues. We must put our nursing house in order regarding differentiation and move on to other pressing issues on the nursing agenda.

Immediate problems confront us in the education arena as we move into the future. We must deal more effectively with mobility. Styles (1979) notes that a striking shift in the ANA's position occurred in the 1978 convention, when resolution 3, in support of accessible, high-quality mobility options, was passed. This resolution ended the concept of rigid education systems and opened the door to the view of each degree as a stage of academic progress.

This does not imply that any degree program should fail to provide academic integrity, but rather that each must be complete in itself and prepare the individual for meaningful employment in its stated occupation field. It does imply that individuals who wish to set new goals and realize new ambitions— hallmarks of a pluralistic society—should be encouraged.

Current trends show a staggering increase in those seeking mobility. Between 1975 and 1984, the number of nurses enrolled in baccalaureate nursing programs increased from 3,763 to 10,000 individuals annually (Hart & Sharp, 1986). Practical nurses are entering associate degree and baccalaureate programs in increasing numbers as well.

It has been said that by the year 2000 there will be a serious undersupply of baccalaureate- and master's-prepared nurses and an oversupply of associate degree nurses. Mobility options will alter that future significantly. In a period of declining enrollment, mobilizing students have become a significant applicant pool and provide for an immediate alteration in the "mix." This phenomenon will help to resolve one supply and demand problem, but it will not help with the shortage of individuals choosing nursing as a career.

Increased nurse patient ratios; decreased funding for nursing education; a shift of females to predominently male occupations; the status, pay, and working conditions of nursing; and a declining birth rate continue to contribute to this dilemma. Young men and women and those seeking a career change simply are not drawn to nursing in sufficient numbers. We had been producing nurses in steadily increasing numbers for many years; that is no longer true. The demand for nurses within and beyond the structured setting has been far in excess of supply in more recent years, and declining enrollments will only complicate this situation further. The registered nurse vacancy rate was 13.6 percent in 1986, and it shows no sign of abating (Moccia, 1987). The applicant pool in schools of nursing has declined by 26 percent since 1984, and the decline in graduates is expected to be 15 percent by 1990 (Moccia, 1987). As the demand for nurses increases, the diminishing supply will become critical.

Divisiveness in nursing is a serious contributor to this issue. It is especially damaging to associate degree nursing as long as the future of the ADN nurse's role is perceived by the public to be in jeopardy. We must present to the public a clear image of who and what we are. We must work harder to merge the image of nursing held by the public and that held by the profession. Nursing must project an image that nursing values. We are often our own worst public relations representatives. How can the public value what nursing does not? We must do more to make the public aware of the continued and growing value of the nurse as a care giver and advocate in this new and complex health care system. Certainly many less prepared and untested groups are emerging and marketing themselves as ready and able to meet the needs of the public while nursing engages in internal turf battles.

On the demand side of the shortage issue, we shall have to seek strategies to increase monies available for preparing nurses, as well as strategies to better coordinate and utilize the labor pool available. That brings us full circle, to the need to continue to prepare high-quality technical nurses in programs that are adaptable to a changing environment, without compromising the vital worker Montag envisioned and worked to produce. Their contribution to quality care and to the ability of the professional nurse to realize advanced practice and leadership roles will be critical to a promising future for nursing.

Just as the health care system is changing, so must the system that prepares nurses to interact with that environment. We cannot live in the past or rest in the present. Rather, we must move into the future, with all of its uncertainties. Through unified effort, we can chart that path in a manner that serves to advance nursing and enhance the health care of the public we serve. Let us remember our roots and mission and take pride in our role in the history of nursing. Let us expand the role of the professional nurse to meet the challenges that confront health care, rather than diminish roles within nursing to serve internal visions and to seek short-term solutions to long-term problems. Let us move into our tomorrows confident of our unique role and our continued significance to the health and welfare of this society.

REFERENCES

American Nurses' Association. (1987). *Analysis of membership options, effects on ANA's membership base, finances, programs and services.* Kansas City, MO: Author.

Anderson, B. E. (1966). *Nursing education in community and junior colleges.* Philadelphia: J. B. Lippincott.

Brown, E. L. (1948). *Nursing for the future.* New York: The Russell Sage Foundation.

Bullough, B. (1979). The associate degree: Beginning or end. *Nursing Outlook, 27* (5), 324–328.

DeBack, V. (1986). Competencies of associate and professional nurses. In *Looking beyond the entry issue: Implications for education and service* (pp. 43–51). New York: National League for Nursing.

Fondiller, S. H. (1986). Licensure and titling in nursing and society. In *Looking beyond the entry issue: Implications for education and service* (pp. 3–19). New York: National League for Nursing.

Hart, S. E., & Sharp, T. G. (1986). Mobility programs for students and faculty. In *Looking beyond the entry issue: Implications for education and service* (pp. 53–66). New York: National League for Nursing.

Mead, M. (1963). Why is education obsolescent? In Gross, R. (Ed.), *The teacher and the taught* (pp. 261–276). New York: Dell.

Moccia, P. (1987). The nature of the nursing shortage: Will crisis become structure? *Journal of nursing and health care, 8* (6), 321–322.

Montag, M. L. (1959). *Community college education for nursing.* New York: McGraw-Hill.

Montag, M. L. (1980). Looking back: Associate degree education in perspective. *Nursing Outlook, 28* (4), 248–250.

National Commission on Nursing Implementation Project. (1987). *An introduction to timeline for transition into the future nursing education system for two categories of nurse and characteristics of professional and technical nurses of the future and their educational programs.* Milwaukee, WI: Author.

National Council of State Boards of Nursing. (1986). *Guidelines on entry into practice: Fact sheet.* Chicago: Author.

Perkins, J. (1983). *Associate degree education: Are the parameters real?* Paper presented at the 1983 regional conference for faculty development in associate degree education, Atlanta, GA.

Primm, P. (1986). Entry into practice: Competency statements for BSN's and ADN's. *Nursing Outlook, 34,* 135–137.

Rines, A. R. (1977). Associate degree education: History, development, and rationale. *Nursing Outlook, 25* (8), 496–501.

Rotokovich, R. (1986). ICON: A model of nursing practice for the future. *Nursing Management, 17* (6), 54–56.

Styles, M. M., & Wilson, H. S. (1979). The third resolution. *Nursing Outlook, 27* (1), 44–47.

Swenson, R. S. (1972). Philosophy of technical nursing and ADN education. In Rasmussen, S. (Ed.), *Technical nursing: Dimensions and dynamics.* Philadelphia: F. A. Davis.

Waters, V. (1965). Distinctions are necessary. *American Journal of Nursing, 65,* 101.

Waters, V., & Limon, S. (1987). *Competencies of the associate degree nurse: Valid definers of entry level nursing practice.* New York: National League for Nursing.

VNA SURVIVAL: WHO'S CALLING THE SHOTS

Gloria Pace King, BS, MBA, RN
President and Chief Executive Officer
The Visiting Nurse Association of Cleveland
Cleveland, OH

I was asked recently by one of my board members whether I thought that visiting nurse associations (VNAs) have learned anything from the interesting and exciting things that our counterparts in the hospital community have been experiencing. I replied with the story of three moose hunters, who happened to be health care administrators.

Three Americans went north of the border for their annual moose hunting expedition and strategic marketing retreat. They were flown into the wilderness in an old, rickety tin goose piloted by a retired Air Force surgeon. Before the pilot left the three hunters, he called them together and said, "Okay, have a great time. Be careful with your weapons. And remember, however successful you may be, we can only take one single moose back as a trophy of the hunt."

The week passed, and the hunters were successful beyond their expectations: each one bagged a moose. The old bush pilot returned, and, of course, each of the three hunters was so proud of his success that he refused to give up his trophy.

"Look," the pilot said, "I told you guys only *one* moose could go back."

"Yeah, yeah," the hunters said. "You told us that last year, then we each paid you 50 bucks and you let us put three moose on the plane. So let's cut the BS and get going."

The pilot scratched the stubble on his chin, evaluated the long- and short-range implications of his action, and said, "Okay. But this year it's going to cost 150 bucks each."

The hunter/administrators paid up, of course, and then spent the next 20 minutes stuffing their prizes and themselves into the sagging fuselage of the of the plane. There was moose crammed into every inch of tin goose.

221

Finally, the pilot fired up the engine and launched the lurching plane into the sky. The plane soared skyward, then groaned, sputtered, and nosedived to earth 100 yards from where it took off.

Slowly the four men disentangled themselves from the heap of twisted metal and moose meat. The first administrator, who had a background in staff education, turned to the second and said, "Well, do you think we've learned anything from this experience?"

"Sure," his companion said. "We paid this guy 150 bucks apiece and got 50 yards further than we did last year."

Apropos of this story, I think VNAs have learned three things from other health care providers. First, you do not solve problems by throwing money at them. Second, pride in achievement must always be kept at arm's length from greed. Third, that if you do not pay close attention to the rules and regulations affecting your activity, you will probably end up a pile of rubble.

VNA HISTORY: A NATIONAL OVERVIEW

Visiting nurse associations are important, effective partners in our nation's health today, just as they were when they first came into being a century ago.

The visiting nurse movement in this country began during the late 19th century, largely as a response to the health care needs of the urban poor in their new industrialized setting. As Buhler-Wilkerson (1985) wrote, "Public health nursing began in the United States as a small undertaking in which a few wealthy women hired one or two nurses to visit the sick poor in their homes." This was certainly the case for most, if not all, VNAs as well.

The creation of a visiting nurse association is well illustrated by the VNA of Boston. Their "Visiting Nurse Association of Boston Time Line" lists the following key dates and achievements:

- 1882–84: Abbie Crowell Howes and Hannah Adam, two members of the Women's Education Association of Boston who were interested in providing nursing care in the homes of the poor, visited Liverpool, England, to learn the work of the Liverpool District Nurses. In 1884, Howes, upon returning from England, began her vigorous campaign to influence physicians and others to embrace the concept of a home nursing service. In particular, she addressed the Boston Dispensary physicians, who had been providing home medical services to Boston's sick poor since 1796.

- 1885: On November 23, Howes received a positive reply from Dr. W. H. H. Hastings of the Boston Dispensary staff.

- 1886: On January 19, Howes assembled a founding committee, chaired by Phebe Adam, to implement the plan for a home nursing service called the Instructive District Nursing Association (IDNA).

- 1886: On February 8, Amelia Hodgkiss made the agency's first visit in the South Cove district with Drs. Buck and Richard of the Boston Dispensary staff.

- 1892: The Children's Hospital requested that an IDNA nurse visit patients discharged from the hospital in their homes. This successful program initiated the concept of "continuity of care." [Apparently this is where the concept originated.]

- 1895: The IDNA nurse covering the Cambridge service area participated in the first use of diptheria antitoxin. It was undertaken with much trepidation, but with successful results.

This chronology shows that even in the last century, VNAs were on the leading edge of medical practice, and it tells us something about where VNAs should be today as well.

The Visiting Nurse Service (VNS) of New York and the VNA of Buffalo were founded at about the same time and have been prominent in the visiting nurse movement ever since. By 1900, there were 25 VNAs in existence throughout the country. According to Buhler-Wilkerson (1987), they provided 24 percent of the in-home nursing care at the time. Buhler-Wilkerson (1985) also states that "by 1910, the majority of the large urban visiting nurse associations had initiated preventive programs for school children, infants, mothers, and patients with tuberculosis." As she notes in a recent article (1987),

> the visiting nurse seemed an irresistible answer to the complex problem of elevating poor families to a more ordered and healthier realm of well-being. The appeal of the visiting nurse was both symbolic and practical. To her wealthy supporters she was "the safest and most practical means of bridging the gulf. . . between the classes and masses." From the perspective of the sick poor, the visiting nurse brought much needed care and relief from the often extreme burdens of illness.

This is still as true today as it was at the turn of the century.

VNA HISTORY: THE CLEVELAND VNA

In an attempt to take the historical perspective somewhat deeper, I will briefly examine the history of my own VNA, the VNA of Cleveland.

The impetus that led to the founding of the Visiting Nurse Association of Cleveland came from nurses themselves. In 1900, the Cleveland Graduate Nurse Association appointed a committee to study district nursing in other cities. The following year, they distributed circulars in the community in the hope of finding someone to foster such a nursing program in Cleveland. A group of young women known as the "Baker's Dozen," who had for some years been interested in welfare work, met with the Graduate Nurse Association and agreed to find ways and means of bringing nursing care to the "sick poor" in their homes. The VNA came into being in 1902 with a board of 30 charter members. When a Superintendent of Nurses was secured, in May 1902, work started from three settlement houses.

By 1905, the VNA had nurses assigned to Rainbow Hospital, Fresh Air Camp, Babies Dispensary in Friendly Inn, Cleveland Maternity Dispensary of St. Luke's Hospital, and Lakeside Hospital Dispensary. At about the same time, a nurse's salary was provided for a while by the Brownie Club of Hathaway Brown School for the inspection of children going to camp from Rainbow Cottage and Fresh Air Camp. Obviously, the close link between VNAs and hospitals that seemed so normal in 1905 is one that we all would like to renew and maintain today.

In 1907, a nurse was requested by and assigned to the Cleveland Hardware Company. Soon, nine other companies had VNA nurses assigned to provide in-workplace health assistance and to make home visits to employees too ill to work—a service that was a forerunner of industrial nursing. I know that most VNAs today are eager to foster the strongest possible relationships with the major employers in their area and with the health care coalitions that these employers have created.

One historical event of note for the Cleveland VNA occurred in 1907, when a prize-winning emblem for the organization was designed by Herman Matzen. The artist based his design on the quotation, "When the desire cometh it is a tree of life (Proverbs 13:12). In 1912, the Board of Trustees presented this emblem to the National Organizaton of Public Health Nursing as a national emblem for public health nursing.

In 1908, a nurse was assigned to the Cleveland Board of Education, and two years later a part-time nurse was assigned to Bratenahl Village schools. These services were a forerunner of modern school nursing programs.

Agency nurses were assigned to the newly opened Western Reserve University Medical School Maternity Dispensary, where they did prenatal and postpartum visits for patients having at-home deliveries. They also assisted in at-home deliveries on a 24-hour on-call basis. This service was continued for 14 years until a shortage of nurses brought it to an end. Remarkably, our VNA did not resume twenty-four hour continuous availability until 1983. I certainly wish that we had continued from 80 years ago. If we had there probably would not be a competitor in town who could come near us.

The VNAs have always been important laboratories for nursing research and for the development of scholarly publications. In 1909, the VNA published the first edition of *The Visiting Nurse Quarterly*. In 1913, the publication was turned over to the National Organization for Public Health Nursing, and in 1918, it became a monthly publication called *Public Health Nurse*.

Our VNA has consistently been involved in the development of nursing policy and practice for the state of Ohio. Even in 1913, the VNA was a charter member of the Central Committee on Public Health Nursing, which considered standards and employment.

Today, VNAs are important partners in the teaching of community health practice to nursing students. In 1937, an affiliation with Frances Payne Bolton School of Nursing was effected to give senior students experience in public health nursing. The Cleveland VNA currently sponsors a scholarship in community health nursing at Bolton School of Nursing. This affiliation has greatly benefited us as well as the students who have worked with us.

Like most VNAs, our agency formed and has maintained affiliations with many key players in the investigation, planning, and growth of our community's health and human services system. The following are some noteworthy achievements:

1. Inspection of nursing homes for the Cuyahoga County Relief Administration;
2. Cooperative study of Tremont Area, a deprived and needy section, where a visiting nurse office was subsequently opened;
3. Cooperation with the Health Council in a nutrition study;
4. Cooperation with the County Child Welfare Board to care for acutely ill children in foster homes;
5. Service to WPA and assistance in nursery schools;
6. Assistance to the Red Cross in the East Ohio Gas Company disaster;
7. An educational program carried out by the Child Health Association for expectant mothers and fathers, which was transferred to VNA and remained an active program from 1947 until December 1977;
8. Assistance to community organizations in a mass chest x-ray survey; and
9. The loan of eight nurse days per week to Cleveland City Hospital during an acute polio emergency.

We are currently part of our community's United Way, participate in the region-wide Federation for Community Planning, and are a member of the Greater Cleveland Hospital Association. These affiliations enable us to be as effective as we can for our community and for ourselves. In 1956, a physical therapy program was established to provide improved physical rehabilitation services to homebound patients. In 1960, we broadened our scope of patient care by undertaking the supervision of Jewish Family Service homemakers assigned to chronically ill persons. Moreover, at the request of the Welfare Federation, we established a Home Care Program on a demonstration basis. The Home Care Program provided selected homebound patients with the full range of health and social services required to meet their diverse and complex needs. These services were arranged for and coordinated by the VNA home care coordinator.

By 1966, after the five-year demonstration period, the Home Care Program had become an integral part of VNA service. In that same year, we, like many VNAs, received our first Medicare certification. Certainly, at the time all of us in the health care field looked on Medicare programs as a godsend; at present, however, we may be justified in wondering if this heavenly institution has not been appropriated by the other side.

A few more key dates are worth noting: In 1969, we received NLN-APHA accreditation. We are very proud of this accreditation, especially since we are still the only Greater Cleveland home care agency accredited by the NLN.

In 1972, a Professional Advisory Committee was appointed to evaluate agency services and community needs and to recommend a direction for agency programs.

In 1978, the VNA and Fairview General Hospital established a Continuing Care Program to ensure that patients being discharged from the hospital (or under its ambulatory care service) would receive needed home care services to improve or maintain their level of health. This was the precursor of a number of VNA hospital–coordinated discharge programs and constituted our first preferred provider agreement.

In 1980, the Ohio Nurses' Association organized the VNA's registered nurses and became their first union for collective bargaining. Naturally, this action had a considerable impact on our agency. Fortunately, we have a very solid working relationship with our nurses, and they and we have continued to work together for the agency's progress.

In 1981, we opened our Hospice Home Care Program, the largest such program in our area. We will seek Medicare certification for this program this year.

In 1983, our board approved and instituted a Medical Advisory Board to provide physicians' counsel on the development and implementation of patient care policies and procedures. That year we also began our own Home Health Aide Program and implemented enterostomal therapy, the first of our high-tech nursing services.

In 1984, we began actively pursuing preferred provider agreements with local hospitals, and by 1985 we had eight hospital contracts, our highpoint to date. At present, we have contracts with five of the approximately 30 hospitals in the Greater Cleveland area.

THE CLEVELAND VNA TODAY

Last year we departed from our traditional medically oriented programs by starting our housekeeping service, Home Neat Home. This service is available to anyone in the community on a fee-for-service basis. Advertising has been targeting the upscale consumer.

This year we will implement full 24-hour private-duty registered nurse care to supplement the round-the-clock practical nurse and home health aide programs we have had since 1983. We have also expanded our core, or regulated, programs into three contiguous counties to the east and west of Cleveland. Soon we will implement a handyman-chore service, which will target midscale to upscale clients, also on a fee-for-service basis.

We have a number of projects under consideration for 1988. On the advice of my administrative staff, I will not detail them here. Suffice it to say that a number of them are likely to put the VNA of Cleveland on the leading edge of home care experimentation and practice, and I am very proud of my staff for taking them on and developing them.

This brief history should serve to illustrate how a more or less typical VNA has grown and developed, over the last 85 years. With this as a background, we can now address the main issue of this paper, namely, who is calling the shots?

WHO IS CALLING THE SHOTS?

I have found that VNAs attempt to be proactive in the development of programs, services, and strategies that anticipate the activity of our rapidly changing health care environment. In all candor, however, for all our efforts to get in front of an evolving reality, we often are and must be responsive to changes dictated from outside the warmth and security of our own strategic plans.

I believe that there are 13 key players who are calling the shots for VNA survival today, and that to ignore the needs, mandates, or even whims of any one of them is to court disaster.

The Patient

The first player in our arena is the patient. The hospital prospective payment systems instituted by government and private payors have caused patients to be discharged "quicker and sicker." Patients need more comprehensive care from and more teaching by their home care providers than they did even two years ago.

Further, patients are desirous of a more holistic structure to their care. Family, diet, exercise, and stress management issues are often raised by patients in even the most elementary and straightforward of care situations. If we add to this the determination among Americans generally to be informed consumers who rightfully demand the whys and wherefores of the care they receive, it is clear that home care providers must be responsive to a new spectrum of patient needs, concerns, and demands.

An important coplayer here is a patient's family or significant other(s), who can have a great impact on the care the patient receives. A cardinal rule in the selling profession is that people do not buy what they need: they buy what they want.

Thus, we may have a situation in which we find 70-year-old children caring for a 90-year-old parent. The comprehensive care plan naturally would take into consideration the potential physical and emotional frailty of all parties involved. However, we may also find a situation in which the caretakers are members of the "sandwich generation," who must care for and nurture their dependent parents as well as their still-at-home children. In such households, the demand may be high for additional services based on convenience and lifestyle. For these cases, it is critical that the VNA provide one-stop shopping for all desired services, from in-hospital private duty care to transportation to companion service and more.

It should be clearly understood that VNAs must see the demands of today's patients and their caregivers as opportunities to explore new markets. These markets are created by desires, by wants, not just by medical needs.

Staff

The second player in our VNA survival game is our own staff. Registered nurses today are definitely career-oriented, seeking an employer who will provide them with a career path that offers ongoing, long-term professional growth and renewal. Today's nurses also demand competitive wages and benefits commensurate with their education, experience, and skills in relation to other professions. These factors may lead to conflict during times of potential retrenchment, such as most home care providers are currently experiencing.

It is important to note that a nationwide nursing shortage is now affecting all health care providers. At one time nursing was the logical career choice for the young person whose aspirations combined a desire to serve and an interest in prospects for advancement. Now, however, many lucrative career alternatives are available to quality candidates.

An illustration of the competitive status of nursing compensation was visible recently in Greater Cleveland. One of the three largest hospitals in the area raised its starting salary and wage scale for registered nurses. Within two weeks, the other two largest hospitals had raised their wage scales above that of the first, which then felt compelled to raise its wage scale again to attain parity with the other two. This compensatory seismic disturbance will doubtless be felt throughout the Cleveland health services system for some time to come.

One final element to be considered here is the unionization of medical staff at all levels, from nurses to aides to companions. Collective bargaining can have a significant impact on the competitive position of any home care provider. It is critical, therefore, to foster an open and forthright working relationship between all parties to a collective bargaining agreement.

The ability to recruit the finest staff possible and to retain that staff by providing fulfilling, rewarding career opportunities is critical to the survival of VNAs today.

Discharge Coordinators

The VNA must always be aware of the needs and desires of the third key player: the discharge coordinator, who can act within a hospital, another inpatient facility, or a physician's office.

The discharge coordinator may be a registered (or other) nurse, a social worker, a medical secretary, or even a temporary office worker. These staff members bring highly variable levels of skills and experience to their activity as referral sources. They also bring a number of preconceptions, and occasionally even misconceptions, about home care and any given home care provider.

It is extremely important that the VNA adapt—as much as is medically prudent for the patient—to the specific needs of these individuals who play such a key role in the referral process.

Educators

Two different types of educators are important to VNA survival today. College and university educators, who train our future nurses and help our current staff to enhance their skills and knowledge, must take into consideration the realities of today's health services system. They must be pragmatic in the teaching of skills that will help their students to be competent caregivers. They also must focus on the future, so that their students are prepared for the techniques and procedures that, though rare now, will soon become commonplace in our rapidly evolving health system. Finally, and perhaps reluctantly, educators must teach the fiscal side of healing. Today's students must understand that quality caregiving is not without cost, and that costs must be compensated. Staff development directors and staff educators are also vital to VNA survival. They must keep themselves, and the agencies they help direct, ahead of the environment. They must endeavor to guard staff competency and quality. In an era of retrenchment, these positions must be nurtured and protected.

Educators, whether in-house or external, contribute a great deal to VNAs' abilities to cope effectively with current medical and social realities. They are also major determinants of whether VNAs will be prepared for the constantly evolving future.

Hospital Administrators

Another key player helping to call the shots for VNAs today is the hospital administrator. It must be stated that the operating style and philosophy of hospital CEOs or administrators can vary greatly from person to person, and often day to day. Candor and a willingness to work hard toward a viable affiliation can be of little value in a home care agency when they are not met with equal honesty and effort from others.

My vice president for patient services recently attended a seminar for hospital administrators. In one workshop he heard the presenter say, "Remember, home health agencies need you more than you need them. Cut whatever deal is good for you and your hospital."

Hospital administrators undoubtedly have their patients' well-being in mind when they negotiate preferred provider agreements. What VNAs must understand is that there is no standard approach to developing and maintaining a solid, stable working relationship with a hospital or its administration: each agreement or attempt is a unique case. A VNA must be persistent in determining the specific needs and wants of any administrator vis-a-vis home care for his or her hospital's patients. The VNA must then be able to demonstrate conclusively why it is the inevitable best choice for that hospital.

Free-Standing Competitors

Perhaps the most interesting player to consider is the competing free-standing home health agency. Whatever one may predict about some future shakeout in the home care field, in Cleveland we have experienced an explosive growth in the number of competitors. In 1980 there were fewer than ten other home care providers in our service area, but today there are more than 40 Medicare-certified agencies in our major county alone.

We who work in VNAs can learn a great deal from our competitors. We can observe them to obtain tips on what to do: how to accomplish niche marketing, how to begin new programs or services quickly and effectively, or how to run a cost-efficient operation. On the other hand, watching our competitors also confirms our feeling that there are some things that we would never do. We would never accept a referral for a service that we do not provide; we would never begin rumors about the financial standing or quality of our competitors; and we would never sanction a case assignment procedure wherein a supervisor would meet with a nurse in a gas station lot, toss her an address, a phone number, and a requested time of visit, and head for the next staff member at the next "drop site." In short, our VNA would never undertake an activity, policy, or procedure that violated our trust as a partner in health to the entire community. I believe that this statement can be made generally for VNAs around the country, but I am not sure that it applies to organizations run by people who have entered home health care as an alternative to operating a motel, an office temporary agency, or a swimming pool cleaning service. At any rate, we watch our competition closely and try to stay as many steps ahead of them as we can.

Joint Commission on Accreditation of Hospitals (JCAH)

One of the newest players in the home care arena is the Joint Commission on Accreditation of Hospitals (JCAH). As more hospitals have opened their own home care programs, it has become natural for JCAH to take an interest in standards for home care. From my perspective, there is some concern that VNAs that had preferred provider or other agreements with hospitals or other JCAH-accredited facilities would also need to be accredited in order for their affiliating hospitals to pass muster with JCAH. For my part, having obtained accreditations from the state and the NLN, I would not look forward to the prospect of undergoing a third, and doubtless rigorous, accreditation procedure.

National League for Nursing (NLN)

One of the most valuable players for the VNA of Cleveland is the NLN itself. We have maintained our standing as an NLN-accredited home care provider. The self-study and review procedure mandated by NLN is extremely valuable for us, in that it forces us to undertake an honest appraisal of everything that we are and hope to be. It allows us, in essence, to compare ourselves to the finest home care providers in the country. We use our NLN accreditation extensively in our marketing efforts and materials, and this strategy has been very effective. We pay close attention to the standards that NLN develops in home care and strive to meet them in all we do.

United Way

A player that is very important to us in Cleveland, but may be less so to other VNAs, is our local United Way. Our United Way is the major source of our indigent care funding. Although we count on United Way dollars to help us care for the needy of our community, we find that our allocation is not keeping pace with the need that we face daily. In 1980, United Way funds represented 21 percent of our budget; in 1987, they represented 12 percent. We understand that our United Way must strive to meet new and emerging community needs, but the "old needs" met by "old-line agencies" have not vanished just because the calendar has moved on.

Our United Way affiliation is also notable here in that it dictates certain constraints upon our ability to raise funds. Thus, we find our indigent care needs outstripping our United Way allocation, but we are not able to approach the community independently to ask it to invest in us and our programs.

There is no question that our United Way funds are vital for meeting critical needs today. There is also no question that a significant increase in allocation is essential, because many needs are currently unmet. Our VNA has chosen to work closely with the United Way to broaden its community outreach efforts, in the hope that a better-educated public will demonstrate substantially increased giving.

Third-Party Payors

A player that may become more critically important over the next few years—if not overnight—is the private third-party payor. The HMOs and PPOs have brought a new game plan to health care delivery. Unfortunately, in prepaid health systems home care is often an afterthought. Further, it is important to remember that a hospital's affiliation with an HMO or PPO can invalidate a preexisting agreement between that hospital and a home care provider. And because group health plans can be extremely cost-conscious, they are unlikely to be moved by the argument that the fees for VNA services include a component for provision of indigent care. Consequently, VNAs must be very attentive to the needs of these relatively new health care consortia.

All VNAs must also be aware of other considerations within the private payer arena. It is safe to say that insurers will no longer pay for all things medical and that consumers must assume risk at a much lower plateau of health services cost. In a time when one's health policy is likely to devote significant space to what is not covered, VNAs must effectively advocate home care as a valuable, cost-efficient health care alternative.

The Media

The media also play a role in calling the shots, in at least a couple of different ways. Investigative reports on health care have touched on home care several times recently. Fairly extensive reports by television stations in Washington, DC, in Cleveland, and nationally have drawn attention to the very real potential for abuse in home care situations. A recent newspaper series in Pittsburgh drew attention to the dismantling of the Medicare benefit and the specter of home care patients left helpless when their care proved nonreimbursable. Unfortunately, such reports, important and valid as they may be, paint all home care providers with the same extremely negative brush.

If these investigative reports are not balanced, within themselves or via editorial response, they can cause needless fear among patients, families, and caregivers. It is infuriating that home care clients are preyed upon by unscrupulous or unqualified providers, but it is tragic that reports of such abuses may prevent the appropriate, effective use of home care services provided by caring, competent professionals. Accordingly, VNAs must be vigorous, forceful, and consistent in their efforts to provide the "good news" about their activities to their media representatives.

The media have also increased in importance, and value, as advertising has become more important in the daily life of our VNA. In Cleveland, there is significant "provider-versus-provider" advertising throughout the entire health delivery system and across all media. Our VNA is committed to effective advertising and marketing and has empowered a competent staff to implement a comprehensive advertising/marketing plan.

An interesting advertising battle has erupted recently in the Cleveland area, where one of the major third-party payors and the local hospital association have waged an acrimonious campaign against each other over the nature and extent of hospital costs. If this particular example is any indicator, health services providers had better be, or become, very clever and knowledgeable in presenting the reasons behind what they do, why they do it, and why it costs what it does.

Power Brokers

The power brokers of any given community are also influential in calling the shots (or, occasionally, missing the call). We recently encountered what we regard as a missed call, when the chairman of the board of trustees of a major Cleveland teaching hospital persuaded his board that the hospital should do its own home care. Our VNA had a long-standing, positive relationship with that hospital. But history, satisfaction with service, and even mutual admiration meant little in the face of one community leader's persistence.

On the other hand, a community's power brokers can also be protective of "their VNA" and can use their influence and expertise to help the VNA stay on top of environmental change in the health field and in the general community. The leadership and guidance that these individuals can bring to VNAs, whether as board members or simply as friends, can be invaluable. They must be cultivated and involved in VNA activities, so that as they call the shots for their community, they ensure that their VNA stays on target but out of the line of fire.

Government

The single most important player calling the shots for VNAs today is, of course, the government—generally the federal government—by virtue of the reimbursement for services that the government may or may not provide.

Federal Perspectives.   The federal government has become visibly concerned with a number of consumer issues that can significantly affect home care. Quality assurance is a hot topic today, and justifiably so. Representative Edward R. Roybal's Quality Assurance Act seeks to protect patients against poor care, neglect, abuse, and exploitation. These are legitimate concerns, and protection may well be necessary, because of the explosive proliferation of home care providers. Although VNAs must, and I believe do lead the way in the development and implementation of comprehensive quality assurance policies and procedures, we must monitor the regulatory process to be sure that the measures being designed do indeed contribute to quality assurance and do not simply encumber providers with another paper chase or administrative waste of time.

The creation of long-term care insurance is another important issue in Washington. Federal support for such care is vital not only to our nation's rapidly increasing elderly population, but also to the functionally impaired of all ages. The specter of acquired immune deficiency syndrome (AIDS) haunts all of us in the caregiving professions and further reinforces the need for effective, nationally funded, long-term care coverage. A new accompaniment to such coverage is the catastrophic care insurance proposed by various parties. At present, the proposals are indeed catastrophic in their failure to include allowances for expanded provision of home care. It should be remembered that VNAs have given long-term care for a century. We should be major players in the development of strategies to meet our nation's emerging health care needs.

Medicare.   As most VNAs, if not most home care providers, can attest, Medicare reimbursement perspectives are a major daily issue for consideration and action. It is difficult to avoid the conclusion that the Medicare benefit is being dismantled. Regulation, interpretations of regulation, and even report form changes occur as though they were timed so as to keep home care providers perpetually off balance. Payment for services provided seems to be capricious at best. The VNA of Cleveland is at present a 100,000-visit-a-year agency. Our case load is 80 percent Medicare. I estimate that we spend nearly $150,000 in salary and benefits annually to staff whose only job is to help prevent denials on the front side or to contest denials on the back. We have seen Medicare payment delayed by as much as two years for denials being reconsidered. The elimination of periodic interim payment (PIP) is considered by most to be inevitable, and the development of prospective payment (home care DRGs) is probably not far away. The present Georgia prospective payment project, in which hospitals are given the prospective payment amount for all services, including home care, can hardly bring Georgia VNAs unmixed delight. I believe very strongly that when the shots are being called in this way, the only option for VNAs is to significantly decrease dependence on Medicare case load.

Indigent Care. Government on all levels is also calling the shots on the provision of indigent care, which has traditionally been important to VNAs. Across-the-board cutbacks for nearly all programs have decreased public funds for the medically indigent. The United Ways in most communities have not been able to completely make up for lost funding. Even when VNAs are given a free hand at fund raising, the competition for private and corporate dollars is fierce. In 1987, the VNA of Cleveland will provide $1 million in indigent care. We believe there is a need for double that amount, but we see no funding sources that will take us anywhere near that level.

It was inevitable, though perhaps unfortunate, that VNAs and other home care providers would become extremely dependent on various sources of government funding. It is likely that nearly all VNAs are actively seeking to distance themselves from the influence of government reimbursement "reconsiderations" by seeking other markets for their services. There is indeed a severe danger that patient needs will be overshadowed by reimbursement considerations, and VNAs are not immune from this deterioration of our health services system.

Given the present state of affairs, I believe that those of us in VNAs must listen very carefully to a diverse and often divergent group of publics, each of which believes that its own needs or wants should be the last word on what a VNA should be and how it should be that. Nevertheless, though I believe that, as a VNA CEO, I should listen carefully, in the end I am the one who runs my agency. In other words, VNAs have their futures in their own hands. By and large, they are competent to ensure viable, even successful, futures.

A VNA SURVIVAL KIT

At the VNA of Cleveland, my staff and I have developed what we like to think of as a "VNA Mind-Set Survival Kit." This survival kit contains the following propositions.

1. The traditional VNA is dead.
   - Indigent care cannot be a VNA's reason for existence.
   - Fraternal feelings about long traditions will not keep a community's VNA alive.
   - Don't be leveraged to do "just a couple of things."
   - Don't just pursue the frail elderly as clients.

2. VNAs should survive.
   - Quality, competence, and commitment to community do have value.
   - We should be able to do home care better than anyone else.

3. VNAs are business.

- A nonprofit corporation is still a corporation.

- The stockholder in our business is our community. We must guard its equity.

- We have no God-given right to exist.

4. VNAs must make sound business decisions.

- Services must be provided according to their potential to sustain themselves financially, or else must be sustained by donations or profitable programs.

- VNA administrations and boards must provide solid financial and managerial expertise.

5. Diversification is good.

- Vertical integration can be beautiful.

- Nontraditional health care and convenience services can help capture clients for traditional home health care. If we provide housekeeping now, they'll think of us for nursing later.

5A. Diversification is good, but look before you leap!

- Don't joint venture, or do corporate reorganization, or start a hospice just because everyone else is doing it.

- Make your own sound business decisions on the basis of your corporate goals, opportunities, environment, abilities, and limitations.

What survival can mean in today's competitive health care marketplace is illustrated by my favorite health care story.

Two CEOs from competing home care agencies went on a deep woods camping trip together. No sooner had they set up their tent and arranged their campsite when they heard a tremendous crashing, thrashing, and roaring in the underbrush.

They poked their heads out of the tent, and saw a 16-foot grizzly bear charging directly toward them. The first CEO, who happened to run a VNA, calmly sat down in the tent, removed her hiking boots, and laced on a pair of running shoes. "Are you crazy?" her companion shouted. "You can't outrun that bear!"

The VNA exec serenely opened the flap to the tent and replied, "I don't have to outrun the bear. I only have to outrun *you!*"

REFERENCES

Buhler-Wilkerson, K. (1985). Public health nursing: In sickness or in health? *American Journal of Public Health, 75* (10), 1155–1161.

Buhler-Wilkerson, K. (1987). Left carrying the bag: Experiments in visiting nursing, 1877–1909. *Nursing Research, 36* (1), 42–45.

THE ROAD TO SUCCESS:
THE NURSE-RUN BUSINESS

Janet A. Moll, MS, RN
Geriatric Nurse Practitioner
Partner, Nursing Associates
Vice President, Institute of Gerontic Nursing
Dallas, TX

The time is ripe for the nurse entrepreneur. There is a new emphasis on wellness and prevention in our society and an eagerness among consumers to have access to nursing professionals with this specialized knowledge. Nurses and schools of nursing are opening nurse-managed centers to provide direct care to clients. Nurses are self-employed as consultants to hospitals, nursing homes, schools of nursing, and numerous other institutions.

To be a nurse entrepreneur in private practice is hard work. My partner, Dolores Alford, and I opened our practice in 1974 after one year of study and preparation. All the income generated by the practice went back into the business for over five years. In 1974, private practice for nurses was a very new idea, and it was more difficult to begin a private practice than it would be now. We persevered, and today, 13 years later, our practice has become a model for primary nursing care of older adults. The practice has expanded to four satellite clinic locations at senior centers and retirement housing around the Dallas–Fort Worth metroplex.

In 1985, we established what will be the nonprofit arm of Nursing Associates: The Institute of Gerontic Nursing, Inc. The Institute will offer education, consultation, and research in gerontologic nursing. This will allow Nursing Associates, a partnership, to focus on direct services to older adults and consultation on private practice for nurses.

Our practice has outlived the statistics for the small business. The *Wall Street Journal* (January, 1982) reports that over 600,000 new businesses are started each year and that within one year approximately 50 percent are gone and within five years 80 percent have folded. There is a 90 to 95 percent failure rate for the average small business.

What are the factors that contributed to our success? One asset was the different strengths and experiences of each partner. The adage that two heads are better than one is actually true. We capitalized our own business and were never in debt. We were also able to support ourselves outside our practice while getting our business going. More than anything else, both of us had a commitment to and belief in what we were doing.

SHOULD YOU START YOUR OWN BUSINESS?

There are both advantages and disadvantages to having your own practice or business. Heading the list of advantages is the control over decision making and the creative freedom available. Profits are tied to the performance of the business, not just to cost of living. Moreover, as your own boss, you cannot be fired or laid off. The pride in owning and managing your own business is also a big plus.

There are also many disadvantages that come with owning a small business. Financially, there is a risk of the loss of your investment and the fluctuation of your income. A regular paycheck may not exist for some time. A certain amount of pressure is created because of the total responsibility for meeting deadlines, paying bills, salaries, and taxes; and working long hours. Finally, gone are the days of paid sick leave, holidays, vacations, coinsurance plans, and the ability to leave your job behind (Kishel & Kishel, 1981).

Many people underestimate the personal traits required to withstand the rigors of small business ownership. A prospective small business person should be able to answer yes to all of the following questions (Small Business Administration, 1973).

- Are you a self starter?
- Is your health excellent?
- Can you make decisions?
- Can you lead others?
- Can you take responsibility?

Plan to spend six months to one year on preparing to go into business. Set goals to accomplish each month. Make your goals measurable—for instance, "Month 1: contact the Small Business Administration for information, review books on starting a small business." Project the date on which you plan to open your business. Determine when your business should break even financially and when you should begin showing a profit.

DETERMINE TYPE OF BUSINESS

It is very important to be able to describe all the services you have to offer. Write your services down to help ascertain your target audience and facilitate the design of a brochure. Are you a consultant, an educator, or a direct service provider? The more flexible you are, the stronger your economic base. For instance, if you plan to provide direct services to older adults, as we do, your specialty provides an excellent opportunity to offer educational programs or workshops to professionals and consumers. You may also want to market yourself as a consultant to certain agencies. As a rule, a master's degree in a specialty field is required if you wish to offer these kinds of services.

Consider selecting a name for your business that provides recognition and an identity for your business. Contact your accountant or lawyer regarding registering your name with the proper authorities.

DETERMINING OFFICE LOCATION

The first decision to be made is whether you will have a home office or an outside office. A home office is certainly less costly and can work very well for the consultant or beginning entrepreneur. It is best, however, to check with your accountant to be sure you meet the tax requirements for a home office. An outside office is generally preferable: it presents a more professional business image, and many people are more productive in this setting. There are many ways of keeping expenses low, such as sharing an office with others, and office rental packages.

The location of the outside office may be determined by the demographics in different areas and the people you wish to serve, or by the costs of office space in different areas. Be sure the exterior and interior of the building project the image you want: warmth and success, without ostentation.

STRUCTURING THE BUSINESS

There are three legal forms of business: sole proprietorship, partnership, and corporation. Sole proprietorship makes up 75 percent of all businesses. Partnership is available for two or more persons, and a written partnership agreement should be signed. The corporation is an artificial being that has an existence separate from that of the owners and therefore is taxed. The cost of incorporating runs from $500 to $1,500. Discuss the best choice for your business with your accountant and lawyer. Study the advantages and disadvantages of each structure in books on starting a small business, so that you are prepared to discuss the issue.

Most people agree that it is best to start out in the simplest business structure possible, and then incorporate when the business has grown to a point where this becomes necessary or when advised by your attorney (Moskowitz & Griffith, 1984).

RECORD KEEPING

Consult an accountant regarding setting up and maintaining the financial records that must be kept. Obtaining advice early can prevent problems later. Proper records must be kept on all income received and expenses incurred. These records will serve to control overhead expenses and cash flow and meet tax and regulatory requirements. An accountant can advise you on the type of bookkeeping and accounting system to utilize.

A bookkeeper or accountant can be paid to maintain your books if you do not wish to maintain them yourself. Maintaining your records on a computer, if one is available, is desirable. Be sure you understand the principles behind the bookkeeping records. Bookkeeping courses are generally available through the Small Business Administration, community colleges, and adult education courses. You should also learn to read balance sheets and income statements (Riccardi & Dayani, 1982). A balance sheet is a summary of the business's assets, liabilities, and capital on a given day. An income statement is a summary of the business's income and expenses during a specific period. These financial statements will be requested if you apply for a loan, whether for personal or professional reasons.

You will also want to establish administrative records to help the business run smoothly. Even if there are only two partners in the practice, you will want to establish certain office policies to ensure continuity and efficiency in running the business. These policies may address the following: personnel policies; billing, credit and collections; or standard forms utilized in the practice.

It is important to keep a record of all appointments, deadlines, time utilized on a project, and secretarial time utilized. The office should maintain one master calendar in addition to each person's individual calendar. A record of business mileage should also be kept by each person for tax purposes (Pearson, 1984).

Records also must be maintained on each client served, whether you are providing direct care or serving as a consultant. Develop an admission or intake form for each new client. The clinical forms or contract utilized must be decided on and standardized. The record-keeping and filing system must be designed for maintaining accurate and confidential records. Utilize a consultant in your area of practice to help you in this area. This will prevent you from "reinventing the wheel."

FINANCIAL CONSIDERATIONS

Part of the planning process involves estimating the amount of money needed to sustain your business for the first six to 12 months. This will be the initial investment. You will need to calculate the average monthly overhead to operate your business. Since most people underestimate how much it costs to run a business, it is recommended that you overestimate and build a cushion. The areas to consider are identified in Table 1.

Potential contacts for obtaining capital include banks, credit unions, savings and loan associations, the Small Business Administration, and partners. It is desirable to be financially able to capitalize the business yourself or with a partner, to avoid a loan and incurring a debt. It is even more desirable if you are able to support yourself part-time, while you work at getting your practice off the ground.

ESTABLISHING FEES

Perhaps the most difficult area for nurse entrepreneurs is placing a price on their services. Many nurse consultants are guilty of undercharging because of inadequate calculation of the expenses of their overhead. Your fees must be competitive, yet designed to be profitable. Determine what the competition (if there is any) is charging and what the market is paying for services such as yours.

There are many ways of establishing your fees. You must first determine your overhead or indirect expenses. If you are a consultant, you may use a daily, or per diem, billing rate. Douglas Gray (1986) suggests a formula to calculate your daily billing rate. Once your daily billing rate is established, your hourly rate is calculated by dividing by eight hours. Most consultants prefer a minimum number of hours (four to six) for contract work, for reasons of cost-effectiveness. A client is generally charged more per hour if less time is used. The client is also generally billed for travel and telephone time and any direct expenses.

Be sure to put your consultant fees in writing to provide a guideline for working with clients. You may elect to send clients a copy of your consultant fees so that there is a clear understanding of the billing policies. Be sure to consider such areas as preparing bibliographies, continuing education applications, and allowing audiotaping or videotaping of any presentations. Remember, you and your talents are the only commodity you have to market.

An hourly fee calculation can also be used if you are providing direct nursing care to clients. Most nursing care, such as teaching, counseling, or assessment, takes time and can be charged to the client according to the actual or average time required to provide the care.

Some consultants give a client a fixed price quotation for a certain project. This flat rate builds in the cost of direct labor, expenses, and a profit margin. There are several ways of establishing your fees. Decide ahead of time if the fee will be negotiable and plan for that factor.

MARKETING

The key to success in the business world is the ability to market your services. In many cases, it is helpful to develop a brochure that explains the services you have to offer and provides background material on you as a professional. This brochure can become your best marketing tool. Whether you give a talk to a consumer group, or mail the brochure, you leave something in the person's hands to refer back to when they need you. You may want to consult someone on the design and development of your brochure. Your stationery and business cards should be designed at the same time, so that typestyle and design remain consistent.

The next step is writing your press release to announce the opening of your business or practice. This release, perhaps accompanied by your brochure, should go to a list of persons or groups you have identified in your professional field and the media. Do not hesitate sending this information to national organizations, journals, newspapers, and television and radio stations. We were interviewed by several newspapers and also were on several radio talk shows. It is still intriguing to both nursing colleagues and lay people that a nurse has a private practice.

Memberships in your professional and specialty organizations are very important. Networking with professional colleagues helps establish a basis for referrals. Be vocal about your activities in your practice or business; you must be your own press agent.

Of course, your goal is to be paid for your services, but many times it helps to donate some free time. Donating time to boards or community groups or actually providing some direct care can begin to put your name in front of people. Providing free talks to consumer or professional groups on your specialty area (as long as you can distribute your brochure!) helps to market your services.

Advertising in journals, directories, or newspapers must be done according to professional guidelines. We have not found these methods useful in marketing our services; yet every presentation we ever made to a consumer group yielded at least one referral.

LEGAL CONSIDERATIONS

Meet with a lawyer and an insurance agent early in your planning stages. They can advise you on your legal concerns and insurance needs. Use your lawyer to help establish standard contract forms or letters. Your lawyer can also review potential contracts, office policies, or insurance policies and advise you on them.

You will need two or more insurance agents because of the diversity of your insurance needs. Discuss your practice with your professional insurance carrier agent, and let him or her advise you on the need for malpractice insurance in addition to your personal policy. You will also need to talk with an insurance agent about the following kinds of insurance: general liability, auto liability, fire and theft, disability, life and health, and workmen's compensation. The costs of the various kinds of insurance are then added to your overhead expenses (Braddock & Sawyer, 1985).

GETTING MORE HELP

Two of your most helpful advisors when you are establishing your business will be your lawyer and your accountant. Build a good relationship with both early in your planning stages, and let them guide you as needed. A business or professional advisor is also helpful, if available. Our 13 years of success as nurse entrepreneurs has attracted individual nurses and colleges of nursing for advice and consultation. We have helped nurses with an idea in its inception or critiqued material once it was developed. It is helpful to consult with people in business in a similar field. You can gain a lot from their years of experience.

The Small Business Administration (SBA) should also be high on your list of contacts. One phone call will provide you with pamphlets and brochures designed for the person contemplating starting a small business (SBA, 1978, 1984a, 1984b). Workshops or seminars are also available through the SBA. Colleges and universities offer courses that may be useful, such as accounting. Libraries and bookstores have numerous books on how to start and manage a small business and how to run a consulting business.

The local Chamber of Commerce is a good contact, since most Chambers are eager to promote local businesses. Trade and professional associations can also help you promote your business. Consider joining an organization such as the National Association of Women Business Owners as a way of networking with other entrepreneurs.

Becoming a nurse entrepreneur is not for everyone. Yet the nurse who chooses to venture into the world of small business will have opportunities for growth and experiences that he or she will never have as an employee. Being in business for yourself is challenging and rewarding, and even invigorating. If nurse entrepreneurship is for you, it is an opportunity not to be missed.

Table 1.   Overhead Expense Categories

Office rental	Insurance
Telephone	Legal fees
Answering service	Accounting fees
Office supplies	Entertainment
Clinical supplies	Auto expense
Postage	Taxes: payroll
Printing/copying	federal
Books and subscriptions	other
Repairs/maintenance	Salaries
Equipment/furniture	Professional memberships

REFERENCES

Braddock, B., & Sawyer, D. (1985). Becoming an independent consultant: Essentials to consider. *Nursing Economics, 3,* 332–335.

Gray, D. (1985). *Start and run a profitable consulting business.* British Columbia, Canada: International Self-Counsel Press.

Kishel, G., & Kishel, P. (1981). *How to start, run, and stay in business.* New York: John Wiley and Sons.

Moskowitz, L., & Griffith, H. (1984). To incorporate or not to incorporate. *Nursing Economics, 1,* 246–249.

Pearson, L. (1984). Self-employment income: Professional fees and tax considerations. *Nursing Economics, 2,* 52–56.

Riccardi, B., & Dayani, E. (1982). *The nurse entrepreneur.* Virginia: Reston.

Small Business Administration. (1973). Starting and managing a small business of your own. Washington, DC: Government Printing Office.

Small Business Administration. (1978). Marketing for small business (Publication No. 89). Washington, DC: Government Printing Office.

Small Business Administration. (1984a). Learning about your market (Publication No. 4.019). Washington, DC: Government Printing Office.

Small Business Administration. (1984b). Starting an independent consulting practice (Publication No. 204). Washington, DC: Government Printing Office.

Wall Street Journal. (1982, January). Small businesses. 29.

THE NURSING SUPPLY:
WHAT DO THE DATA SUGGEST?

Peri Rosenfeld, PhD
Director of Research
National League for Nursing
New York, NY

Earlier articles in this volume have addressed some of the key issues in contemporary health care and nursing: the aging American population, the introduction of prospective payment for hospital care of Medicare patients, and the movement to alternative health care delivery systems.

These social, economic, and political trends clearly affect nursing, and hence nursing education as well. Numerous important questions arise, but I will restrict myself to a single major one, namely, Are nursing educational programs meeting the needs of the changing health care environment? More specifically, in terms of manpower (or womanpower), are there sufficient supplies of variously prepared nurses to meet the demands of the current health care climate?

Using data from the National League for Nursing's annual survey of nursing educational programs—a comprehensive study of *all* nursing programs (see Figure 1)—I will present a series of graphs that reflect the historical trends in nursing education. These past and present data will provide a backdrop against which the nursing school population, and ultimately the nursing supply, can be discussed (National League for Nursing, 1987).

ENROLLMENTS AND GRADUATIONS

That nursing school enrollments have been declining is known. The year 1984 marked the beginning of this downward trend, and the 1986 enrollments have dipped to just over 200,000 (see Figure 2). This figure represents a loss of over 50,000 students since 1983. The last time enrollments were at the 200,000 point was in the early 1970s (1971–1972). Over the past decade and a half, diploma enrollments fell by more than half, associate degree enrollments increased by one third, and generic baccalaureate enrollments have gone up and down since the late 1970s and are now about 10 percent higher than they were then. By the way, associate degree programs enrollments were steadily increasing until their peak in 1983. The 1986 figure represents an 18 percent drop from that peak.

The declining enrollments have, not surprisingly, resulted in fewer graduates of basic registered nurse programs in 1986 (see Figure 3). The year 1985 marked the all-time high for the number of new graduates from basic RN programs: 82,075. The 1986 figure, however, represents a 2.5 percent drop, and we expect deeper drops in the next few years. The current 1986 graduation figure of 80,000 is approximately 7,000 higher than that of ten years ago. Like diploma enrollments, diploma graduations fell by half over the past decade; associate degree graduations increased by 10,000. Basic bachelor of science in nursing (BSN) graduations actually increased over the past two years; however, decreases are expected to materialize next year.

BACCALAUREATE PROGRAMS

Fortunately, the news is not all bad: the number of registered nurses returning for baccalaureate degrees has been increasing steadily and dramatically over the past decade. In fact, the RN enrollment in BSN programs jumped from 19,000 in 1970 to 45,000 in 1986—an increase of 135 percent in a decade. Similarly, RN graduations from baccalaureate programs have grown by 123 percent over the past ten years; from 4,737 to over 10,000 (see Figure 4). Although registered nurse graduations from baccalaureate programs have stabilized in the last few years, this can be explained by the fact that these students are most likely to attend part-time and hence graduate in varying lengths of time.

The Department of Health and Human Services' fifth report to Congress on the status of America's health personnel considers two categories of RNs: one contains diploma-prepared and associate degree-prepared nurses, and the other contains nurses with a baccalaureate or a higher degree (US DHHS, 1986). The supply of diploma and associate degree nurses may be ''in balance'' (according to this report), but the supply of baccalaureate–prepared nurses and nurses with higher degrees is not.

As several of the preceding articles have indicated, health delivery settings such as community health and public health, which have traditionally been the realm of BSN graduates, are growing rapidly. Hence, although the number of BSN-prepared nurses is increasing, it cannot catch up to the current and projected requirements. In short, despite disagreements over the DHHS's projection of the future supply of registered nurses, no one could deny that the demand for nurses with advanced degrees will not be satisfied in the future. Even the DHHS projects a shortfall of at least 600,000 baccalaureate and higher-degree nurses by the year 2000.

HIGHER-DEGREE PROGRAMS

As early as 1983, the Institute for Medicine study on nursing personnel concluded that the need for graduate-prepared nurses—specifically, nurses with master's degrees or doctorates—is not being met, and the gap is widening (Institute of Medicine, 1983). Nurse administrators, researchers, clinical specialists, and others trained at the graduate level are very much in demand, and despite the continued growth in master's and doctoral programs (see Figures 5 and 6), it is unlikely that the supply will satisfy the demand.

Master's Programs

To counteract any tendency to pessimism, it is worth pointing out that the number of master's enrollments has grown by 40 percent since 1980 alone (see Figure 7). The mushrooming of graduate programs is encouraging, and we have every reason to believe that these trends will continue. Since the majority of master's students attend part-time, the length of time before graduation varies. Nonetheless, master's graduations have grown by over 30 percent in the last five years!

Doctoral Programs

Finally, let us look briefly at nursing doctoral programs. New programs continue to burst on the scene: only 14 such programs existed in 1976, but now there are 38 operating programs, with over 1,800 enrollees (see Figure 8). From the vantage point of the nursing school faculty and administration, graduate nursing education heralds good tidings and hope. Unfortunately, as mentioned above, even these exciting figures will probably not satisfy the future need for graduate-prepared nurses.

CONCLUSIONS

What do these data tell us about the current nursing shortage and future nursing supply?

First, while the current number of basic registered nurse graduates is still relatively high in comparison to past years, this will probably not continue for much longer. The numbers of basic RNs will stabilize and possibly drop. Ultimately this will affect supply. However, baccalaureate and graduate level nurses will remain in short supply for the forseeable future.

The changing health care delivery system requires a better educated nurse, one who provides autonomous care in the community and hospital, makes "on the spot" decisions, supervises practical nurses and represents nursing to hospital administration, runs her own business, and does research at the National Institutes of Health.

Ironically, both the current shortage and the nursing opportunities available are consequences of the changing health care delivery system. The truth is that nursing is full of attractive career choices. Our mission is to continue to bring this truth to the public.

REFERENCES

Institute of Medicine. (1983). *Nursing and Nursing Education: Public Policies and Private Actions.* Washington, DC: National Academy Press.

National League for Nursing. (1987). *Nursing Student Census With Policy Implications 1984–1986,* New York: Author.

U.S. Department of Health & Human Services. (1986). *Fifth Report to the President Congress on the Status of Health Personnel in the U.S.*

Figure 1. Basic RN Programs, 1960–1986

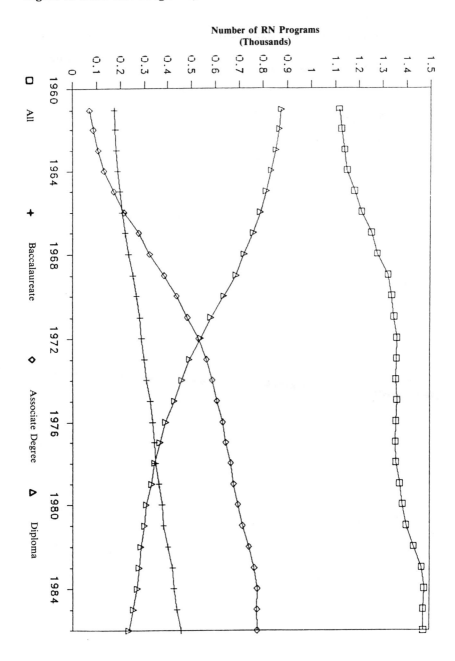

Figure 2. Enrollments, 1960–1986

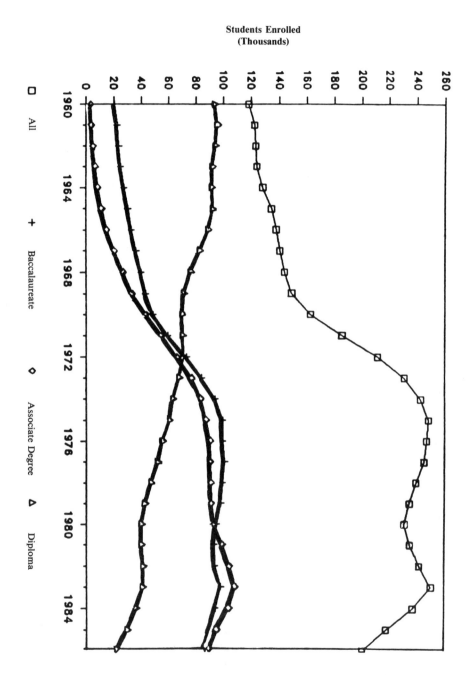

Figure 3. Graduations, 1960–1986

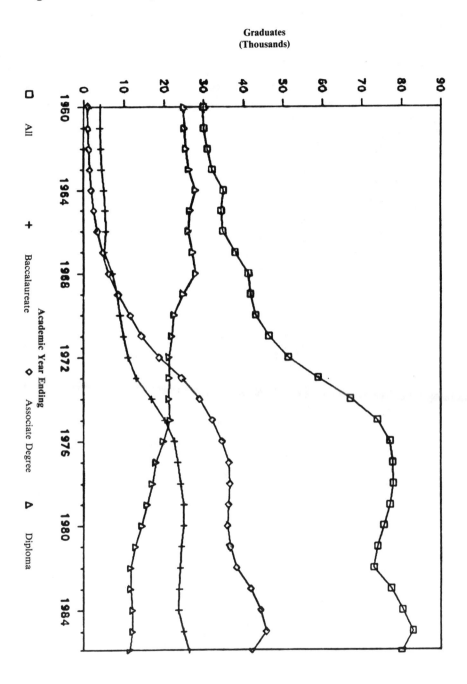

Graduates
(Thousands)

Peri Rosenfeld

Figure 4. RN Graduations from Baccalaureate Programs

Students Graduating
(Thousands)

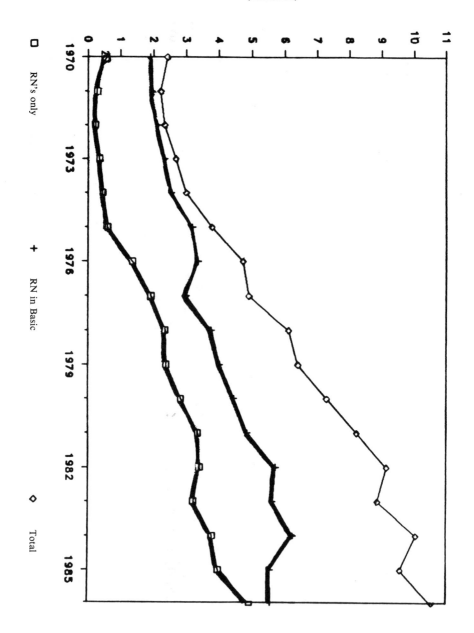

Figure 5. Growth of Nursing Master's Programs

Number of Master's Programs

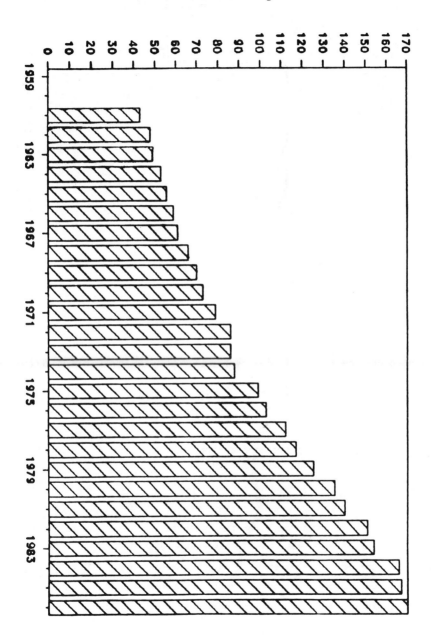

Figure 6. Growth of Nursing Doctoral Programs

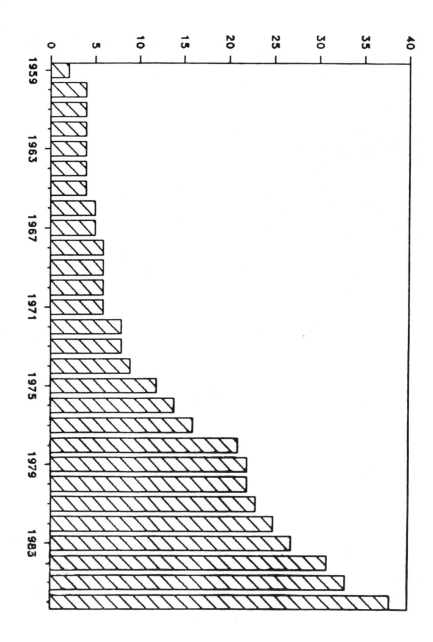

Number of Doctoral Programs

Figure 7. RN Enrollments in and Graduations from Master's Programs

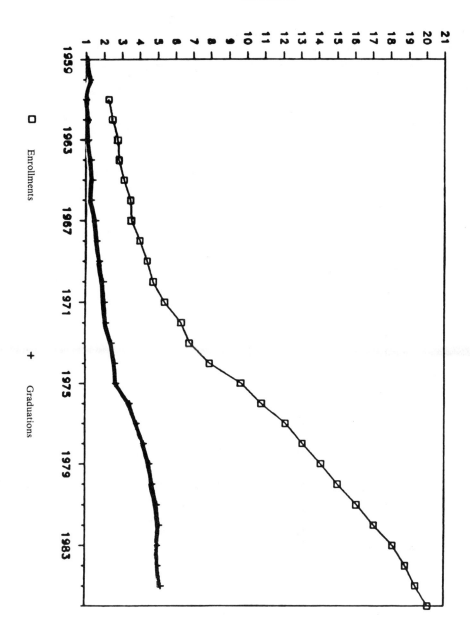

Students Enrolled or Graduated
(Thousands)

Figure 8. RN Enrollments in and Graduations from Doctoral Programs

Students Enrolled or Graduated
(Thousands)

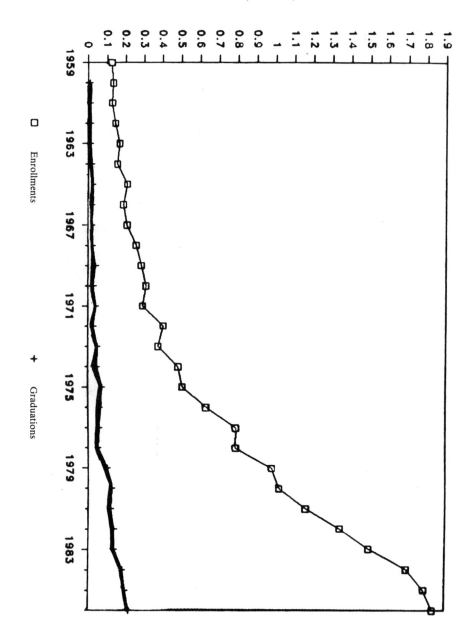